FOR THOSE WHO SEARCH . . .

The program outlined in The Low Blood Sugar Handbook is for you. It is an optimum lifestyle not only for functional hypoglycemics (low blood sugar sufferers), but also for those suffering from premenstrual syndrome (PMS) and everyone else who desires a healthy and productive life.

Women who suffer from PMS often have low blood sugar. Once the blood sugar is stabilized, the PMS can be dealt with more effectively.

This book is written by low blood sugar sufferers rather than by a medical person since only sufferers have the insight into dealing with the everyday situations of low blood sugar. After working with hundreds of hypoglycemics, Edward and Patricia Krimmel have articulated the things that only sufferers can know. They give the clear, practical and complete advice you need for understanding and dealing with the everyday nitty-gritty of low blood sugar.

The chapters of the book deal with such practical matters as being able to identify if you have low blood sugar, what it is, how serious it is and what to do if you have low blood sugar.

The KRIMMEL PROGRAM is covered in detail. Its four dimensions are:

- Food ethic
- Exercise
- Fun & laughter
- Sleep, rest & relaxation

A fifth dimension is found in chapters 5, 6, 8, and 9. The information is unique to this handbook. Only through the application of the fifth dimension, can the low blood sugar sufferer get total value from the other 4 dimensions.

Low blood sugar is a personal affair. Only through personal initiative can it be controlled. There is no medication or "cure all" for it. Only through the proper program and understanding your body chemistry can this condition be controlled.

Having low blood sugar diagnosed and treated properly is too often near impossible. This is the major reason the Krimmels have written The Low Blood Sugar Handbook.

> If you're willing to spend enough time
> And put out enough effort
> You can solve every problem
>
> *John Brown, In Memory of his Friendship*

Here's what users are saying about The Low Blood Sugar Handbook:

"I have just read your handbook and immediately put myself on the program. After two weeks I am feeling well enough to spend time in my office and have utmost hope that I can finally get may life back together."

Kalamazoo, MI

"The Hand book has been a life-saver for me. I believe my friend suffers from LBS and wants to borrow my book so please send me one as soon as possible so I can pass it on to my friend."

Danielson, CT

"Thank you for your wonderful book, 'The Low Blood Sugar Handbook'. It is a tremendous help to me and to others I know who have read it as it offers a wholistic and insightful understanding of hypoglycemia along with a balanced and supportive recovery program. I am heartily grateful for your efforts."

Cambridge, MA

"Thank you so much for your wonderful book, I really think it helped save my life! I am feeling so much better I can't even believe it!" After stopping all caffeine, sugar and artificial sweeteners, I could feel the difference in 2 days. Mostly I feel much calmer, like I'm not stretched to my maximum tolerance at all times. I'm nice to my poor husband, as I don't 'snap' on him as I used to, and things at work are now on a more even keel. I just returned from vacation and for once I wasn't a total nervous wreck about travel."

Phoenixville, PA

"Your handbook has been such a help to me. I've been off sugar for two weeks now and the improvement with myself is almost too good to be true."

Syracuse, NY

"Thank you for writing the Low Blood Sugar Handbook. I can't even begin to tell you how it has changed my life. I have recommended it to several of my friends and relatives."

Mastic Beach, NY

"I am so grateful for your book . . . I've read every book on the subject of low blood sugar and yours is the best."

Kettering, OH

"I have found your handbook and cookbook to be invaluable assets to my daily well-being. I thank you greatly for them."

Idaho Falls, ID

"The handbook has been my survival kit for the past year. I've lost 20 lbs. since I've been off sugar, white flour etc. Everyone says I look great."

Quebec, Canada

"Your handbook has been my bible since the day I purchased it. It has been a gift from Heaven."

Indian Rocks Beach, FL

"Your books have done wonders for me and I want this information passed along to a friend so she can learn about the condition. She is also searching for answers and solutions to her problem."

Brooklyn, NY

"Thank you for the life-saving services you are doing for LBS sufferers. My son feels good for the first time in years after following your handbook plan. I thank you from the bottom of my heart."

Hillsboro, OR

"Your Low Blood Sugar Cookbook has been a true life saver! I now wish to order your Handbook and Cookbook for my daughter."

Grove City, OH

"Congratulations on your informative and all inclusive low blood sugar book. A friend loaned me hers, so please send me one for myself. Not only was your book enjoyable to read, but it answered so many questions that I have had for years."

Williston, ND

"Both my doctor and I have been amazed at my incredible improvement. To think that I suffered for so many years. Also, I've always had such problems with weight gain and now I am able to maintain an ideal weight and still enjoy eating."

Orange, CA

"I am a recovering substance abuser and have found the program in your handbook most helpful and beneficial. Since stabilizing my blood sugar, I no longer have anxiety and tremors. Thank you! I tell everyone at the AA meetings to get your handbook and follow the program."

Wilson, TX

"I bought your handbook, read it through thoroughly, and had my whole family follow the program. We can't believe how much it has improved all of our lives. All of us have better moods, no headaches, no tiredness and my children's grades have even improved. Thank you, thank you, thank you!"

Indian Wells, AZ

We dedicate this book:

To everyone who is interested in their well-being and especially to those who suffer and are told there is nothing wrong with them or it's all in their head; to those who are being treated for a condition but are not getting better; to those who have been diagnosed as hypoglycemic but have not been able to stabilize their blood sugar.

And to those brave people who are willing to think and talk about faulty body chemistry being the root of many health and social problems.

And to our Parents for being the fountainhead of our lives and spirits.

In memory of *Al* and *Bob*.

To Charles, Ethel, Nancy, Tom, Hugh and Jerry with the joys and memories of the past and future.

Ed & Pat Krimmel

ACKNOWLEDGEMENTS

To Dr. Mae Leone for having expressed love and concern for a fellow human being and showing us that the light at the end of a tunnel can be knowledge, not a locomotive.

To the low blood sugar sufferers who allowed us to work with them.

Ronald Bermon, Lewis Creskoff, James Duffy and Homey Writer for your help.

To Michael Molloy for his kindness and generosity.

Dr. Harvey Ross, thank you for being you.

Charles, thank you for your kindness and consideration while we were writing the book.

Eswari Pattela, thank you for allowing Charles to draw on your love and the warmth of your home during the writing of the original manuscript.

Last but not forgotten, all the doctors who did not diagnose the condition, for they gave us the opportunity to suffer, struggle and evolve into stronger, wiser and more enriched persons. Suffering and struggling are the essence of evolution, with a little time and a dash of space required.

A RECIPE

Always climb a mountain one step at a time.
Question who you are and why.
Allow yourself enough time and energy.
Start at the base and seldom look at the top.
Keep your hope and desire high and your expectations low.
You will find every step a reward to the most important person
in the world . . . yourself

Ed Krimmel

Inch by inch everything is a cinch!

Dr. Robert Schuller
The Hour of Power

THE
LOW BLOOD SUGAR
HANDBOOK

You Don't Have To Suffer . . .

Edward A. Krimmel
Patricia T. Krimmel

Preface by
Harvey M. Ross M. D.

Art & Design Editor
Charles A. Krimmel

FRANKLIN PUBLISHERS

Box 1338
Bryn Mawr, PA 19010

This book is not intended to replace or substitute in any way the services of a physician. Any application of the recommendations set forth in the following pages is at the reader's discretion and sole risk.

CONTENTS

PREFACE

By Harvey M. Ross, M. D.

Dr. Ross is a Diplomat of the American Board of Psychiatry & Neurology practicing in Los Angeles, California. A founding member and past president of the Academy of Orthomolecular Psychiatry; on the Board of Trustees, The Huxley Institute for Bio-social Research. He is author of Fighting Depression and co-author of Hypoglycemia: The Disease Your Doctor Won't Treat, The Executive Success Diet and The Mood Control Diet.

The time it takes to diagnose a broken leg may be measured in minutes or hours. The time it takes to diagnose hypoglycemia from first symptoms to final diagnosis is usually measured in months and years. Considering the severity of emotional and physical symptoms experienced by those with hypoglycemia, and the time it takes to make the proper diagnosis, the enormity of the problem in terms of waste may be appreciated. Wasted years, unfulfilled goals, impossible interpersonal relationships, lack of professional attainments are but part of the price paid by those with undiagnosed hypoglycemia. The remainder of payment in terms of misery is made by those who are close to the person with hypoglycemia; the family; the friends. They too suffer.

Hypoglycemia is a cause of misery which can be eliminated. An informed public, and informed medical community is all that is needed to treat this condition successfully. The first step taken by most people is to seek medical help. When medical help is not found or when the wrong attitude or wrong answers are given, the search soon ends and individuals begin to rely on themselves.

The Krimmels have provided an excellent guide to those who find they must treat themselves, as well as to those who wish to find and work with a physician. A close adherence to the program which they outline will result in improvement in most cases of nonorganically caused hypoglycemia.

All the ills of man are not related to hypoglycemia. But there is an unfortunate group of individuals who suffer from fatigue, depressions, irritability, confusion and some physical symptoms who are told year after year by their physicians, "All your tests are normal; there isn't anything wrong with you." Between the covers of this book this group may find the important answers which are necessary for a healthy and productive life.

Harvey M. Ross, M.D.
Los Angeles, California

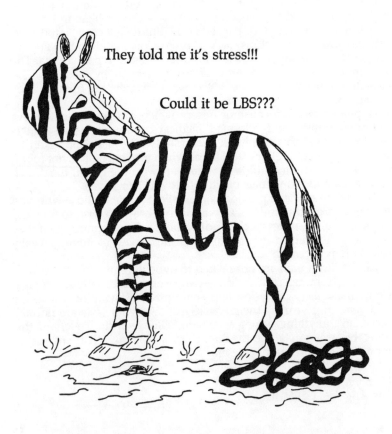

INTRODUCTION

The revised edition is a result of new and improved concepts developed from talking with thousands of low blood sugar sufferers who have bought our books over the years. We wish to extend our appreciation to all those who have shared with us how their lives have improved by following the Krimmel Program in the handbook.

A higher number of people are beginning to take personal responsibility for their own well-being by learning how their bodies function and what is needed for them to function properly.

No longer do hypoglycemics have to be held hostage because they can't find out what is causing their problems. Through reading and studying they are discovering that what they put into their bodies can cause their lives to be disrupted and erratic or calm and controllable.

The word has gotten out that the proper food is often much more beneficial to our bodies than medications.

Even women with premenstrual syndrome often have trouble with hypoglycemia, states Dr. Ronald Norris, M.D., faculty member of Tufts University School of Medicine, Boston, Mass.

Throughout history headaches, depression, alcoholism and sleep problems have been considered as being caused by something other than a body chemistry imbalance. Until recent years the alcoholic was considered to have a character flaw.

Today's research is finding that the 11 million alcoholics,[1] the 36 million depressed persons,[2] the over 100 million suffering with headaches[3] and the 50 odd million with sleep problems[4] are often suffering with a body chemistry problem, which can be improved and sometimes even corrected by taking in the proper foods and their bodies being cared for with tender loving care (exercise, rest and relaxation, and fun and laughter).

Only recently is low blood sugar being recognized as the shadow behind many commonly known problems—many experts working with alcoholics believe the majority, if not all, alcoholics have low blood sugar; a great number of patients with mental conditions have improved immensely after being diagnosed and treated for low blood

1. Alcohol, Health and Research World, Vol. 13, No. 1, 1989.
2. Office of Scientific Information, National Institute of Mental Health
3. National Headache Foundation, 1991
4. Department of Health and Human Services 1990

sugar; several institutions which work with juvenile offenders have tested them for low blood sugar and found a high percentage have low blood sugar.

Aggressive behavior is another area where hypoglycemia shows up. Probably the most dramatic example of this is represented in the studies by Ralph Bolton, an ethnographer. He studied the Qolla, an Andean subculture near Peru, who have a culture with considerable violence and aggression. This is the direct opposite of what their moral code demands, which is charity, compassion and cooperation with all men. So why are they aggressive and violent? Mr. Bolton found a high rate, 55%, of the men he tested had hypoglycemia. Eleven of the 13 most aggressive men in the group had hypoglycemia.

Dare we chance to think that hypoglycemia may be a contributing factor to the high incidence of crime and social problems in the United States?

The primary reason this book has been written is that I am a hypoglycemic (Low Blood Sugar sufferer) and my wife and I are anxious to share the many insights we have gained from living with the condition over the years. Although there are fine books written about hypoglycemia, to our knowledge this is the first to be written by a hypoglycemic. Our book is not so much about hypoglycemia as it is about the everyday nitty-gritty of living with the condition. We tell you the things you should and can do to end your suffering.

The insights we discuss in this book have been developed over years of personal experience. We have tested and retested the methods, not only on me but on other people we have helped to understand and regulate their own hypoglycemia.

On a scale of 1–10 for hypoglycemia severity, with 10 being the most severe, I would rate myself a 8½–9. Before my hypoglycemia was regulated I regularly experienced approximately 40 of the common symptoms of the condition. Now that I am regulated by following the program we have worked out and outlined in this book, I would rate myself a 1 because of the infrequent occurrence of a few of the listed symptoms. Most times these few symptoms occur, it is because I am only human and eat something that tastes good to my tongue but isn't good for my body chemistry. It's the old battle of pain and pleasure that all hypoglycemic victims eventually have to face and deal with. At least now I know why I have the various symptoms and how to deal with them. Having these insights has given me the opportunity to enjoy a very beautiful life. We hope the insights will afford you a better life too.

The program outlined in this book is an optimum lifestyle for not only hypoglycemics, but for everyone who desires a heatlhy and productive life. Naturally it's called the Krimmel Program.

The book is our contribution to the ultimate dream: that one day low blood sugar (hypoglycemia) and all other body chemistry problems will enjoy more credibility, research funding and treatment by nutrition rather than just by medication.

Had it not been for books on hypoglycemia we would still be wandering and staggering through the orthodox medical maze, looking for an answer to the many symptoms I was displaying. Only through the books did I learn what was really wrong with me. Now that I have a free mind and a healthy spirit my wife and I are able to make our contribution to the social fabric which helped us.

Because of the many people we met who told us about their low blood sugar condition and difficulties in getting suitable information, we decided to put our ideas on paper so we could help people more effectively.

We thank those who have given us their sincere encouragement.

So here it is, *your personal handbook,* the means by which you can readily establish whether or not you are hypoglycemic and the specifics of what to do and what not to do. If you find yourself using the material in our book on a day to day basis, then we have done our job well.

We made a special effort to use a level of language that would be complementary to the subject and at the same time be folksy and easily understood by the lay individual.

It is very important that your family and friends read this book so they will be able to understand hypoglycemia and how it affects all of you. Then they can be supportive and helpful.

God bless, and we love you too.

Ed & Pat Krimmel

The authors encourage you to share with them any questions or insights you may have. A great amount of work still needs to be done in the study of low blood sugar and its effects. If an answer is desired, include a stamped, self addressed envelope. Please write to us c/o:

Franklin Publishers
P.O. Box 1338
Bryn Mawr, Pa. 19010

COMMUNITY SUPPORT GROUP

If interested in having a self help support group started in your community or locating one already established, mail your name, address and phone number to: Franklin Publishers, Box 1338, Bryn Mawr, PA 19010. Include a self addressed, stamped envelope.

SUFFERERS BEWARE!!!

Be sure to use the whole wheel, not just half

It is imperative that the information in this book, *especialy chapters 5, 6, 8 and 9,* be kept ever present for immediate recall and use. We, the authors, literally spent thousands of hours learning, conceptualizing and drafting the tools of this handbook. All the information we worked so hard to deliver is not helping you if you only read the book once and then put it aside, thinking you'll remember what to do or lend it to someone else.

Remember, this is a handbook. It is to be used daily, read *again and again and again to help you retain the concepts so you can use them to regulate your blood sugar.* Even we have to keep reading material about LBS in order to stay sharp—*and we wrote the handbook!*

If you want a friend or relaitve to have a copy of the handbook, *we will mail them a copy . . . autographed.* See order form in back of book.

NEWSLETTER! NEWSLETTER! NEWSLETTER!

How would you like to receive current information in the world of body chemistry, nutrition, biochemistry, LBS, PMS, well-being, and so on? Send a self addressed, stamped envelope to: Franklin Publishers, Box 1338, Bryn Mawr, PA 19010.

Chapter 1

COULD THIS BE YOU?

My spirit was willing but my body just didn't seem to have the get up and go it should have. For years I had been telling doctors how I felt but they would simply say I was in great shape and that there wasn't anything wrong, just snap out of it.

Not until I finally discovered I had low blood sugar did I get some insight into what was really wrong with me. Now I can finally understand why I had such a variety of complaints. I had approximately 40 of the symptoms listed below. Why don't you review the list and see what your score is.

A very common reaction by most people when first reviewing the symptom list is to say, "Gee, I've had all or most of these things wrong with me or happen to me". We say in response, "True, but how often and for how long of a duration?"

Bear in mind, no one knows for certain what the ideal is in respect to how a person should feel. It's as vague as a shadow on a wall. But rest assured, if you don't already know, there are some people who never suffer the vast majority, if any, of the symptoms listed below.

Later in the book you will have a reason to review the symptom list again, but for now it suffices to do just a cursory review for your own insight.

Remember while reviewing the list to reflect for a moment and try to make a concise evaluation. It can be difficult to try to make words fit your feelings and experiences. But do your best and give some gut responses and some reflected ones where needed. Don't be hesitant to use a dictionary to be able to get more color and meaning to the symptoms listed.

A word of caution, symptoms alone are not enough to determine whether you have low blood sugar; they are merely one of the tools you should plan to use. Everyone has a few of these symptoms occasionally. But if you have some of these symptoms frequently or always you can suspect that you may have low blood sugar (LBS).

SYMPTOMS

Tiredness
Headaches
Drowsiness
Concentration problems
Irritability
Sleeping difficulties
Dizziness
Anxiety
Forgetfulness
Visual disturbances
Depression
Fainting/Blackouts
Nightmares
Digestive problems
Aching eye sockets
Lack of sex drive
Impotence
Indecisiveness
Heart palpitations
Internal trembling
Mental confusion
Undue sweating
Bad breath
Antisocial behavior
Asocial behavior
Unsocial behavior
Gasping for breath
Obesity
Restlessness
Back ache and muscle pain
Sneezing
Skin Tags

Cold hands and/or feet
Nervousness
Exhaustion
Shortness of breath
Temper outbursts
Sensitivity to light
Sensitivity to noise
Allergies
Muscle pains
Phobias (fears)
Crying spells
Negative thoughts and attitudes
Feeling of going mad, insane
Suicidal thoughts or tendencies
Staggering
Craving for sweets
Unnecessary and excessive
    worrying
Mood swings (Dr. Jekyll & Mr.
    Hyde)
Waking up tired and exhausted
Arms and legs or body hurt when
    first rising in a.m.
Feel best after 7 p.m.
Sighing and yawning
Convulsions with no known cause
Premenstrual tension
"Motor Mouth" (constant talking)
Alcoholism
Accident prone
Family history of diabetes or low
    blood sugar

THE LOST SOUL AND THE ALERT PATIENT

The symptoms you have indicate that something is wrong. Your body is sending you messages through these symptoms, it's the only form of language the body has. The alert patient is the key to health treatment and results. The better able you are to tell a doctor how you feel, the better he is able to treat you.

You say you have done this and the doctor says you are in great shape, he can't find anything wrong. You gave him your money, he smiled and you left with your pack of symptoms still on your back. Or worse yet, you have been told continually that "it's all in your head" or "why don't you grow up" or you are sent to a psychiatrist.

You may have been treated without results for other conditions which low blood sugar mimics. Many low blood sugar sufferers wander like lost souls from doctor to doctor, year in and year out, before being properly diagnosed. We have coined the phrase the *Lost Soul Syndrome* for these wanderers.

Bear in mind that proper diagnosis of low blood sugar takes a tremendous amount of time, interest and a physician who understands the concepts in depth. And one who is willing to give credibility to the existence of LBS. Like most professions, the medical camp is followed by too many doctors who are overworked, uninterested, uncreative, overpaid and in addition simply don't believe that LBS is a problem. Perhaps your biggest task will be trying to locate a physician who does give credibility to the existence of LBS and has an adequate background and an in depth understanding of its ramifications.

Many physicians will say they are concerned and understanding but they are not. Subsequently the safest thing you can do before going to any physician is to be adequately schooled on the subject of LBS so you will know whether the physician has an in depth working and treating knowledge of LBS. It only takes an hour to learn the "buzz" words but it takes total interest and dedication to really help the LBS sufferer.

Once you locate a physician it may be beneficial for a support person to go with you when you see the physician. The support person may prove very helpful in giving some additional refinements about you to the physician. It may even be helpful to have the support person work with you in locating a doctor. Low blood sugar effects the brain and its thinking processes, therefore get all the supportive help you can.

MISDIAGNOSIS OF LOW BLOOD SUGAR

It's painful enough to have LBS and not be able to have it diagnosed, but it's even worse having it misdiagnosed as another condition. In that case you may be given medications that don't help your LBS condition and could even make it worse. As long as it's misdiagnosed there is no way for you to get better. Eventually you are likely to become demoralized and have your faith in the medical profession eroded. Instances of misdiagnosis by one degree or another have occurred probably more than once to every LBS victim. Four specific reasons this occurs too frequently are:

1. Symptoms of low blood sugar are similar to those of many other conditions.
2. Low blood sugar is not accepted as a common medical condition and is not understood by a large number of physicians.
3. Low blood sugar is a body chemistry condition very much tied in with nutrition and most physicians have a limited knowledge of, and interest in, nutrition. Happily though, some are beginning to take an interest in how nutrition and health are interrelated.

4. The diagnosing of LBS requires creative medical thinking. Many physicians are bright academic test takers but are very low in creative thinking.

Following is a list of some of the more common misdiagnosis given to LBS individuals:

Neurosis	Menopause
Diabetes	Alcoholism
Depression	Sun stroke
Schizophrenia	Parkinson's syndrome
Rheumatic fever	Hypochondriac
Migraine	Chronic bronchial asthma
Nerves	Senility
Allergy	Rheumatoid arthritis

Some of the informal comments often used by doctors and others in hope of whipping a LBS person into a turnabout are:

1. Why don't you grow up?
2. When are you going to snap out of it?
3. It's all in your head.
4. What's wrong with you?
5. If only you could cry, you would be all right.
6. How much longer are you going to act like this?
7. There is nothing wrong with you, all of your tests are negative.
8. Think positive.

Perhaps one or more of the above statements strikes a familiar chord. I hope the recall brings you a smile rather than a smirk. My favorite is Number 5. I'll never forget the period in my life when it was said to me.

CASE HISTORIES—
REFLECTIONS OF THOSE PAYING THE PRICE

The following are case histories of myself and some of the LBS sufferers we have worked with over the years. The names of individuals and organizations have been changed to protect their privacy, and any resemblance to persons living or dead is coincidental.

In working with these individuals we encouraged them to read various books and articles on Low Blood Sugar and to talk with other low blood sugar sufferers. Most of the people we have worked with have required 15 to 25 hours of personal counseling to develop a clear picture of the concepts that must be used to maintain a proper blood sugar level. Very often with low blood sugar—you will discover if you haven't already—the small concepts are just as important as the large. But no concept is worth anything unless it is used faithfully.

We have found case histories to be invaluable to LBS victims. Case histories afford a quick and handy reference point-of-view to the condition. The authors hope these histories prove valuable to you too. If nothing else, you will know you're not suffering alone.

Author's Case History

Perhaps you know the song "What a Difference a Day Makes"—well let me tell you about what a difference a person can make. Meeting Mae Leone, the proprietor of a health food store in North Palm Beach, Florida, was probably the best thing that's ever happened to me. After having talked with me for only a few minutes she suggested I buy a book about hypoglycemia. My first reaction was that she was giving me a sales pitch but since the book was only $1.75 I bought it. It has turned out to be the most important purchase I have ever made, and to think I was going to be "EL CHEAPO" and not buy the book. I get chills when I think of all the thousands upon thousands of dollars I have given to the medical camp and received nothing in return but platitudes and hocus-pocus.

When I got home I sat down with the book and began reading. After a couple of pages I let out a whoop and told my wife that this was what I had been telling all the doctors I had ever seen. Here it was, printed right on the pages, all my symptoms and the way I felt; fatigue, nervousness, mood swings, sweating, dizziness, headaches, difficulty with concentration, uncontrollable yawning, irritability, low physical energy, poor coordination, drowsy during the day and restless and unable to sleep at night, vision difficulties, etc. Finally here was something that related to me and my suffering.

I had spent the vast majority of my life feeling as if I had one foot on an ice cube and the other on a banana peel. But I can now say with great relief that my life is completely composed 99% of the time. Years ago little would I have believed that a combination of the proper food, exercise, rest and fun could have saved me from a life of ice cubes and banana peels. I am provoked when I think of all the times I responded negatively when hearing, "You are what you eat." The difference in what you eat certainly does make a difference in how you feel and function. Oh the hells of cultural barriers.

Finally after 45 years of a constant display of hypoglycemia symptoms, I was able to figure out what was wrong with me. However, this was only accomplished after my wife and I had read and studied extensively about hypoglycemia and body chemistry. And by the way, I prayed too. *And did I pray!* My prayers were surely answered—someone reached out to me and gave me some time, thought and consideration. Thank you God and Mae Leone and Pat.

Let me start at the beginning . . . As an infant I apparently cried most of the time, at least that is the impression I have from some of the old family stories.

When I was an infant it was common for junk men to knock at the door asking for rags, papers and scrap metal. One day when the junk man came to our door, he said to my 6 year old brother, "Ask your mother if she has any junk today." My brother came back to the junk man and said, "We don't have any junk today but I have a baby brother who cries all the time, you can have him."

Quite possibly I had low blood sugar even as an infant, however there is no way to know and it doesn't much matter now, so we will leave it lie.

As a child I remember suffering from frequent and severe knee joint pains, headaches, shortness of breath and constant tiredness. Looking back it seems I was always in and out of the medical maze of services. I was diagnosed by a cardiac specialist as having rheumatic fever, a diagnosis that must have been wrong since I have no residual heart involvement as an adult.

I can remember awakening almost nightly with the leg pains and crying. My mother rubbed my legs with Ben-Gay until I finally fell asleep again. These leg pains continued into my early twenties. When telling the doctors, which seemed like thousands of times, about these pains they would always ask about the joint pains in the rest of my body, to which I would reply that I had no other joint pains. This would confuse them to such a point that they would almost insist on my saying yes I did have the pains in my elbows and other joints. However, I never surrendered to their logic by saying I had other joint pains. The doctors never went any further in considering that my condition might be anything other than their first opinion, rheumatic fever.

Due to the rheumatic fever diagnosis I was frequently kept home from school to rest for weeks at a time. Also I was not allowed to participate in sports. And during all of this time I had the so-called luxury of the classic "Apple Pie" Mom, "enjoying" homemade: puddings, pies, cakes, muffins, candies, preserves and root beer. Although Mom had good intentions, she was really loading me with sugar and white flour which probably gave rise to my symptoms. However, in my mother's case there cannot be guilt where there was no knowledge.

While in grammar school I can remember how my eyes would feel as if they were going to the top and back of my head. Often I would walk around as if I were punched out or in a daze. Usually I didn't mention these feelings to my parents because I felt what was the use, since I was doctoring all the time anyway. Besides I wasn't sophisticated enough to have the insight into just how I did feel. And how did I know everyone else didn't feel this way since I had always felt this way. I just knew I didn't like the way I felt, it was sometimes like a twilight zone—there but not there. Anyway, in order to explain how you feel you need to use your brain and my brain was very often shut down. Often I would cause some disturbance in class and the excitement of being scolded or whatever would stimulate me and pick me up, thereby making me feel better and I'd enjoy the relief.

Even though I had a high I.Q. and was a high achiever in non-academic settings, my school work suffered seriously because I couldn't concentrate for very long, and was restless and sometimes fell asleep in class. Reading was my biggest problem, probably because of my difficulty with concentration and focusing on small print. And taking a test was an almost impossible task. Even when I knew the material I would often draw a blank trying to answer the questions. I survived by cheating and being a good talker in class discussions. I dared not bring home a failing grade or my father would have severely punished me. (Looking back, I suspect my father was also a hypoglycemic sufferer—he sure had a collection of the symptoms.)

As I look back upon my youth and remember my struggles, I often wonder how I survived. After school during my teens I worked in a variety of jobs, one being in a pet shop, home of the original Docktor's Pet Center. I remember very vividly on various occasions when I would knock items over or drop them which would give cause to my own embarrassment as well as to the owner's annoyance. One day I even leaned on the glass of an aquarium that I had just repaired. I normally would never have leaned on glass but I was so exhausted and I couldn't think clearly. The glass broke and I was cut severely on my wrist.

Other times I would be so exhausted that I would go to the second floor of the shop and lie down on the floor and fall asleep. On Saturday mornings I was barely able to lift my feet to walk to the shop. It was the same feeling I had walking to school during the week. Usually, once I got where I was going the activity would apparently stimulate me and I could function adequately for a while.

I didn't realize it at the time, but now know naps and food would have revived me. My poor performance was offset by my high productivity and my otherwise conscientious efforts when I was feeling up to par. Looking back I must have often been living off my glands rather than food.

As I grew older my symptoms increased and I continually went to doctors trying to find out why I was suffering. No matter what I said or how I said it to the doctor, I was invariably told I was in great shape and probably would live to be a hundred since I had such low blood pressure.

I was a mailman when I was in the Army, what a great job—but more important it was just perfect for me. I could go into my office every day and close the door as if I wasn't there. I would put my head down on the desk and go to sleep for about one or two hours. I just couldn't keep up, I'd get so beat out. While in the Service I made various attempts to find out what was wrong, again to no avail.

Sometimes I get so angry when I think of all the doctors I went to over the many years and got the same mickey mouse story of how there was nothing wrong with me and I would shell out my money with nothing to show for it. One doctor even put me on dexedrine (uppers) and had it not have been for a conscientious pharmacist I would possibly have gotten hooked, since they did make me feel great. But they were not solving the cause, only treating the effect.

On three separate occasions during my early life (8, 15 and 20 years of age) I passed out. Each of these occasions occurred during the summer months and I was the only one to pass out although there were other people present. Each time I was seen by a doctor but no significance was given to the incident. It was only rationalized away in particular to the context in which it occurred. Looking back it may very well have been another dimension of my low blood sugar—since blacking out occurs frequently to LBS sufferers.

Some additional symptoms which had surfaced by this time were: cold hands and feet—so severe that when swimming in the ocean or during cold winter weather my fingers and toes would turn white and ache so badly that I would be near tears; severe irritability—felt as if my brain was always in a vice and I was falling off the lip of stability; sensitivity to light—I usually wore sunglasses during the day to prevent my eyes from hurting; sensitivity to noise—loud noises would scratch at and short circuit my nerves; loss of peripheral vision—sometimes when driving I would lose sight of the center line; anxiety—felt as if my stomach was being wrenched and twisted; tender eye balls—they would hurt and feel as if they had pressure on them. The burden of the symptoms very often caused a great strain on my social, work and family relationships.

Often I wanted to participate in various events but would hold myself in check in fear of unleashing my various symptoms. Even though I did not relate to my symptoms formally, I developed an insight in relation to how I was affected in various circumstances. Subsequently I developed a "laid back" style of dealing with situations in order to avoid excessive stress. Goodness knows how much more productive and rewarding my early years might have been had I known then what I know now. But that's all in the past.

I was given the nickname "sleepy" by some of my coworkers at a small machine shop even though I was a very productive, conscientious and congenial worker. I would often have severe bouts of sleepiness and exhaustion—to the extent that I could barely stay on my feet. At these times I would often fall asleep in any convenient location, even standing up.

While working for Campbell's soup I would fall asleep everyday at about 10:30 a.m. and 2:30 p.m. I tried everything but I couldn't stay awake. I worked in the accounting department and often my manager would be doing some work with me and I'd go to sleep right in his presence. No matter what I'd try, nothing kept me awake. Fortunately I eventually found employment that as long as I fulfilled my responsibilities I wasn't tied down to any specific hours.

I wanted to go to college so my G.I. bill would not go to waste. But remembering how difficult and frustrating school had been, I didn't see how it was possible. Nevertheless, being the tenacious creature that I am, I took the college entrance exam and got shot down. However, I was still determined, so I made an appointment with the head administrator of the school I wanted to attend and was able to persuade him to let me enroll. I started off with two evening courses, Political Science I and College English I. I eventually dropped both courses because I couldn't keep up. The next semester I took two other courses and stuck with them.

The lectures and discussions in college were pure joy, while most of the rest of the activities were a painful struggle.

However, the academic struggle was not as severe as it had been during my early years in school. Unbeknownst to me at the time, 7 p.m. and after is *magic time* for many hypoglycemics. For some reason or another many low blood sugar sufferers tend to feel significantly better during those hours. This often can be their most organized and productive time. I fared so much better during the evening that often I would say in jest that I must have evolved from the cat family since I was a nocturnal creature. It was probably due to this factor that after six years I was able to graduate from St. Joseph's University in Philadelphia, Pa. with my degree in Social Science and a minor in Economics.

Up to the time I was 35 I had unconsciously developed a very structured lifestyle. Then I did a complete turn about, I left my job of 13 years, got married, and traveled the U.S. for three months. This is when problems really began to ripen. I thought I had troubles before, but they were nothing compared to what lay ahead. In retrospect it seems this complete change of lifestyle caused a major increase in stress which led to a great increase of symptoms. Within a short time I felt as if all four of my tires had been shot out and I was riding around on my rims.

Almost immediately I began having additional symptoms, and the ones I had had became much more severe. Within three months of being married I was talking about getting a divorce—Oh the hells of low blood sugar, when you don't know you've got it, you keep looking for scapegoats to whip! My mood swings became more and more frequent and severe and I was getting a little paranoid along with a feeling of increased anxiety. Although I have never abused my wife physically, I would verbally attack her often in my fits of rage, which in some ways were perhaps more vicious and cruel than physical abuse—Oh, the hells of low blood sugar!

Throughout this period my employment was sporadic. Eight months was the longest time I spent at one job.

In December, 1970, I began sneezing with what I thought was a cold or virus. I sneezed and I sneezed and I sneezed. My nose ran and ran and ran discharging a clear fluid. It seemed endless. I would even wake up in the middle of the night sneezing. My G.P. sent me to allergists, one who told me if only I could cry I would be all right. Another said I was allergic to dust, pork and horse hair. So we thoroughly scoured the house, and avoided pork and horse hair. And still I sneezed. The allergist said he didn't know what was wrong and couldn't help me, but if I ever found out what was wrong to let him know. Eight years later I called him and told him what had been wrong with me and he was so indifferent that I wanted to climb through the phone and strangle him.

Then I went to the ears, nose and throat doctors who eventually convinced me to have my deviated septum repaired. That costly operation was supposed to solve the sneezing—needless to say it didn't. So much for another group of medical trips!

By this time we decided the sneezing must be caused by air pollution since we lived in the city and air pollution was supposed to be affecting everything in the early 1970's. So we sold our house and moved to Ocean City, New Jersey on Novemeber 1, 1971. Granted the sneezing decreased but my irritability, mood swings, and noise and light sensitivity, headaches and cold hands and feet increased tremendously.

My wife grew fearful of starting a conversation with me. I would turn on her and attack her verbally because of my constant misinterpretation and twisting of what she had said. I became a real live *Dr. Jekyll and Mr. Hyde* to my primary family. I would suffer tremendous remorse after verbally abusing them for no good reason. I don't know which was worse, the verbal horrors I would create or the horrible remorse I would suffer afterwards for having caused such a calamity and grief.

In Ocean City we bought a large four story, seventeen room property which needed a lot of work. I worked in the real estate business while upgrading the property. My coordination and vision were so poor at times that I was constantly hammering my thumb, rather than the nails. Simple plumbing problems became major difficulties because my brain wasn't functioning efficiently. I remember spending days trying to solve a one hour problem because I couldn't get my thought patterns and concentration glued together.

It's really spooky to be sitting here writing all this down and have the benefit of a clear thinking pattern in contrast to the times I couldn't achieve the simplest things in mechanics or paper work for which I possessed all the talent and ability that was required at the time—Oh the hells of low blood sugar!

Meanwhile, at the real estate office I was slapping the sales out one after the other, hoping my brain would stay glued together until each deal closed. Fortunately I have a high aptitude for sales, providing there is a market. There was a market for about two years and then the bottom dropped out and my morale dropped with it—the oil embargo of '73—'74 hit and the vacation home market crashed. Now the waiting for a prospect to work with would sometimes be days on end, and I started to blame my tiredness and exhaustion on psychological factors. Well—wouldn't you?

Again I started the treadmill of going from doctor to doctor looking for answers. One put me on thyroid medication, another gave me tranquilizers and ritalin, a stimulant. Each of these would have some benefits for a few days and then the side effects would begin. The thyroid medication made me so depressed that I couldn't function, only sit and look at the ocean with my wife beside me because I was so scared of the feelings I was getting. I thought I knew what the word depression meant until I had the side effects of that medication and a whole new dimension was opened up, I was so down that I wouldn't even reflect on how I felt. Needless to say, I didn't continue on that medication for very long.

My next ventures; for six weeks I drove seventy miles to Philadelphia for acupuncture once a week. I felt some relief for the six weeks but it didn't last. In desperation I went to the Mayo Clinic for a "total diagnostic" work up. Their diagnosis was allergic respiratory disease. Some of their recommendations were; not to have more than a five degree temperature difference between bedroom and the rest of the house, never walk around in bare feet, wear a mask over mouth and nose when out in the cold, etc. Needless to say none of these things helped. So much for creative thinking on their part.

Much to my disappointment I later read that even the Mayo Clinic doesn't give complete credibility to hypoglycemia. Oh well, it was just another of the friendly trips that the medical camp sends us on so often.

During the time in Ocean City I felt as if my world was falling apart piece by piece. Most of the time I was so tired that I couldn't even walk a couple of blocks. I had to drive everywhere, and that even drained me to the point I sometimes had difficulty getting out of the car. I stopped driving at night because the on-coming headlights made my eyes feel as if someone was stabbing them with an ice pick. Sleeping became an ordeal rather than a time of peacefulness and healing. It was a constant battle of nightmares and waking up many times throughout the night leaving me exhausted and frustrated.

Our son was born during this time and was the one ray of sunshine in my life. I could hold him and sing to him and forget my misery for a little while.

While in Ocean City we had many visitors. Because my nervous system was so bent out of shape from my low blood sugar I would inevitably blow my cool whenever I felt psychologically crowded. I would walk around as if waiting for the second shoe to drop. This at times led to very strained and tedious situations which years later I would apologize for. Needless to say my list of friends and relatives deserving apologies was quite long.

Particularly offensive to me were technological noises such as stereos, parked cars idling, helicopters overhead, cash registers clanging in restaurants, etc. These types of noises grated on my nerves so badly that I became very tense, my bones felt as if they were going to crack from the tenseness. My eardrums felt as if there was a great pressure on them. I would begin to get defensive and start thinking about what offensive actions I could take. Unfortunately most of these types of noises came from situations out of my control.

No matter how much I hoped for the return of a reliable real estate market, it just wasn't going to happen. Since there didn't seem to be any real future for us in Ocean City and I had a business opportunity at hand in Pennsylvania, we decided to put the house up for sale.

In Ocean City I always felt as if the world was going to fall apart. When we moved to Wayne, Pennsylvania in May, 1975 it was as if the world had come to an end. My low blood sugar symptoms came into full bloom. Not only did I get more symptoms, but my traditional symptoms became more severe. I felt as if I were physically and psychologically in a vise that was slowly being tightened. It had nothing to do with the change of geography although at the time we thought it did. What it was, was a cloudburst of stress that poured down on us and set my nervous system into a tailspin. Within three months of moving to Pennsylvania both of my wife's parents died and my brother died. He was only 46.

I had left Ocean City for the promise of a business partnership. But, two weeks after I had moved, I was informed by my friend that he had formed a partnership with someone else. My daily existence became a life of stress, stress and more stress. Oh the hells of fate being poured on a low blood sugar sufferer. The hand of fate touches everyone but it is especially heavy to a victim of LBS.

I became impossible. Almost every morning I would create a point-less argument with my wife and leave the house screaming at her. My wife was constantly asking me to grow up and to stop acting like a child. My temper tantrums were almost daily and I would use vile profanity at the drop of a hat, which was very much out of character for me. I was intolerant of all situations and by trying not to show the intolerance I constantly put more stress on myself. Where I didn't keep the lid on my intolerance was with my family.

I found myself withdrawing from most outside situations. Coming in contact with other human beings became almost unbearable. But if I had to, however, the ghost of Dr. Jekyll and Mr. Hyde got me through it. I would be the horrible Mr. Hyde with my family but if someone came to visit or while at the office I would switch to Dr. Jekyll. I was glad this happened but I didn't know why it would occur. Here I was, treating my family members with abuse and contempt a good bit of the time, all of it undeserved, and treating outsiders as nice as pie. The confusion of why this was occurring often built a barrier of indifference, or complacency, or hostility, or anger, or frustration etc., between my wife and me. Oh the hells of low blood sugar!

Unbelievable as it may seem, my wife hung in there and kept coping with the situation as well as keeping faith in me. How she ever did it, I can't completely explain. However I do know she read a book that gives her renewed strength. It's the *Holy Bible.*

Again we broke camp and pulled up stakes, headed West still haunted with the thought that air pollution was mostly the cause of my allergy symptoms and giving rise to my severe changes in personality. To both my wife and me the West and Southwest had always represented clean clear air, free of pollution. So—we sold the house, put the furniture in storage, loaded up our station wagon and headed out on April 13, 1976. Our plans were to drive throughout the Southwest and West and choose an area to live.

After much anguish and many, many miles we settled in Boulder City, Nevada. We chose it, thinking that the air must be clean in the Nevada desert. Within a couple of weeks I began to discover that it was not the clean, clear air oasis we had believed and hoped for. A pure case of not being able to judge a town by its looks. The air quality in the Boulder City and Las Vegas area is badly polluted by air blown over from Los Angeles. Boulder City has high levels of ozone, which can't be seen, but severely affects some individuals' respiratory systems. This I learned after I began feeling like I had straps across my chest and difficulty taking deep breaths. I contacted the local health department and spoke with the head administrator who told me that if I was having trouble breathing in May and June I'd better get out of town before July and August. This is because the hydrocarbons from automobile exhausts are converted into ozone when acted upon by sunlight. Since the sunlight is so severe in July and August and there are more cars due to vacations, the ozone levels would increase greatly. Upon hearing this we decided this was not the best area for us.

In retrospect, we now know that this type of situation has negative affects on me only when my blood sugar is not stabilized.

So on July 1, 1976 the furniture went back into storage and we headed for Triangle Park, North Carolina, where the Environmental Protection Agency has its Air Quality Data headquarters. This was not a random exercise, I had contacted U.S. Senator Howard W. Cannon of Nevada who wrote to the agency in my behalf. Subsequently they had sent us a collection of very pertinent and helpful information which led us to decide on living in the Eastern U.S. rather than the Western part. Since we were going East anyway we decided to visit the agency for more specific information on air pollution. We finally decided on locating along the central east coast of Florida.

Near the end of July we rented an efficiency apartment in Port Salerno, Florida, the swordfish capital of the world. It was while we were house hunting and living in the efficiency that my wife said she thought I might have low blood sugar. She knew I should have protein but didn't know I shouldn't have sugar. She would give me eggnog when I felt very tired and it would pick me up for a short time and then, since it had sugar in it, I would slip back down again.

We went to the public library looking for information on low blood sugar—but the cupboard was bare—Oh the hells of low blood sugar and the inefficiency of some public library systems in not supplying adequate information on human body chemistry and personal well being. Anyone for talking about cultural lag?

After we left Nevada, the straps across my chest left, only to be replaced when we reached Florida with severe muscle exhaustion and aches. I would wake up in the morning feeling as if someone had been beating on my arms and body with a baseball bat all night. I felt like crying when getting out of bed due to the muscle pain and frustration. —Oh the hells of low blood sugar!

Again I went to a doctor and this one said I had allergic rhinitis and put me on prednisone to take as needed for the allergy symptoms. It did give me a temporary relief, but who wants to stay on such a dangerous medication? In my opinion the doctor was negligent to prescribe such a medication in such a casual fashion. He didn't do anything about the many other symptoms. I told him at the time that even though I might look as if nothing was wrong with me, I felt like both arms had been ripped off and I was bleeding to death. As I think back it behooves me what doctors are thinking about when patients are trying to convey concepts of undiscernible pain to them. One thing for sure in my opinion, not one of all these doctors up to this point was thinking about me or if they were thinking about me they sure were negligent. Oh the hells of LBS.

On October 1st, 1976 we moved into the house we had bought in Hobe Sound, Florida. It was a few months later that we went to the health food store and bought the book on low blood sugar. I immediately stopped eating sugar, white flour, and all starches and began eating snacks. I soon discovered that if I ate some protein when I was sneezing, the sneezing would stop. Also I learned if I ate sugar or white flour products or waited too long to eat I would begin sneezing. Suddenly, for the first time in what seemed like a million years, I now had what appeared to be a chance. Eureka, we had discovered a pattern to some of the bizzare things that were happening to me. Could this possibly be the key to help solve the rest of my freakish attacks? Needless to say I begged *God, please, please, please, let it be the case.*

To think that just a few weeks earlier I had asked my wife to sit down and talk with me about a decision I felt I had to make. I had reasoned out that possibly I was never going to be able to find the answer to what was wrong with me. A horrible new dimension of the Jekyll-Hyde syndrome was my over reaction to and harsh treatment of my three and a half year old son when he "misbehaved." When I was in a calm and normal state I would remember how I acted and see myself as a pseudo child abuser. This was nightmarish to my reflective mind. This was the straw that was breaking my back—the decision had to be made. The only choice was for me to start living apart from my wife and son so that I would no longer be present to abuse them. After talking to my wife I did something contrary to what had always been my religious ethic and practice. All my life my style was to pray only in thanks. This time I prayed for help. Looking back I wish I had prayed for help many, many, years earlier, but I guess it just wasn't my time. In my opinion, walking into that health food store and receiving the book on low blood sugar was the answer to my prayer, for without that event I would more than likely still be going from doctor to doctor in blind hope that one of them would take enough interest to help me.

Let me take a moment to dramatize the experience of discovering the health food store, because it sure was an experience in serendipity. My wife, son and I would occasionally drive to Palm Beach for a day's outing. A row of new shops was being built in North Palm Beach along the east side of U.S. 1. We couldn't help but notice the name posted across the front of one of the stores, it read NUTRITION

RESEARCH. We wondered what it was. One thought was that it would be a computer service where an individual gives a history of how he feels and what he eats along with a general overview of his lifestyle and any physical problems he might have. From this he would be given a printout analysis of what he could do to improve his eating habits and lifestyle. Of course we tossed a few other ideas around but none as intriguing or as suited to our interests. Nevertheless, we decided we would stop on the way back and check it out. In the late afternoon we pulled up in front of the store and parked. The sun was low in the western sky which gave cause to a very bright glare against the store's front window, so much so that we were not able to peer in. Had we been able to see that it was just another health food store we probably would not have bothered to go in. However, since we could not see in, we opened the door and started in only to stop suddenly when realizing it was a heatlh food store. Fortunately at this point my wife said, "Since we're here, I'll get some whole wheat flour." Just ponder how fickle it was our having gotten into this store—seeing the sign, a name that caught our attention and interest, the time of day we stopped which allowed the sun to glare against the window, not being able to see into the store and my wife deciding to buy some whole wheat flour. Wow, it blows my mind when I contemplate and reflect upon it.

While my wife was looking for the flour, I stood leaning on the counter gasping for breath. Fortunately it was late afternoon, the time when I usually had some of my most active and most severe symptoms such as gasping for air, severe tiredness, irritability, impatience and looking and feeling downright miserable. The proprietor, the lovely person she was, asked me if I was all right. I said, "Yes, I'm O.K., this is just something I've put up with for years." She asked me a few more questions about how I felt and was affected by various things. I sure didn't feel like playing 20 questions at the time, however my Dr. Jekyll came forward and I politely answered the questions—thank goodness I did, for it was at this point that she pointed to a book rack across the store and suggested I buy the red book How To Live With Hypoglycemia, at the top at the rack. Dr. Jekyll took book in hand, looked at the price of $1.75 and thought it would be a good bargain to pay for getting the proprietor off his back. At the time I thought to myself, "Ain't this something, here I am suffering and feeling almost dead and this hungry merchant is selling me a book." At this point Mr. Hyde was at battle with Dr. Jekyll trying to emerge and breathe his wrath on this hungry merchant. It would not have been the first time it happened in similar circumstances, but Jekyll prevailed and thank goodness.

Twenty minutes later we were home and I sat down with the book and began glancing through it—Lo and behold it sounded like they were writing about me. And they were. And I knew it. Right then and there, I screamed to my wife, "Here it is, here it is, exactly what I've been telling all those doctors," I couldn't believe my eyes. With that my wife came rushing in and sat down beside me on the sofa in our living room. Together we excitedly scanned the rest of the book. Needless to say, that day was the last time I had sugar and many other things for a long, long time.

Within a few days I was haunting every health food store and book store for any books relating to low blood sugar. Why not? For a few measly dollars I could enjoy the luxury of reading information and case histories that I could readily identify with. It was as if I was being liberated from a medical bondage, and I was! *Oh God, thank you!*

Within a few weeks we had bought enough books on low blood sugar and body chemistry to stock a small home library. My wife and I spent hours upon hours diligently studying these new concepts. Each day we would add a little more to our knowledge about low blood sugar and try to utilize it. We soon realized that no one author of any of the books told the complete story, each book made its own contribution to the overall picture.

By the end of our second week of following some of the suggestions from the books I began to notice a significant positive change. For the first time in years I began to feel energized and my body wasn't aching most of the time. The cloud began to move away from over my brain and I could hold a conversation with my wife without going into a rage. Also, when I began sneezing I would eat some protein and the sneezing would stop. We soon learned that sneezing probably meant that my blood sugar was dipping. It was as if my body had a language all its own. Also the use of foul language was a pure indication that I needed to eat. Don't get the impression that I was now Little Lord Fauntleroy suddenly—by no means was I totally stabilized. But for the first time I did start to have some positive feelings that my world was starting to become whole again, mostly because now I was beginning to see a relationship between the cause and the effect of my problem. I was so happy, I felt like a child again—not always but at least sometimes.

Having started to make some progress, we thought it would be a good idea to get a glucose tolerance test, since some of the books suggested it was the most reliable way to discover if you really had low blood sugar. The first doctor I saw ordered the test and said my results showed something. Since he didn't know that much about nutrition he referred me to another doctor in his group. This doctor completely poo-pooed the ideas of low blood sugar even when my wife told him how I would feel better after eating protein and staying away from sugar. I can still see him standing there, smirking while he talked down to us and belittled our findings—the quack. His diagnosis was depression and he said I needed to get some self-esteem going for myself. When we returned home we made a graph of my test results and compared them to the criteria in the books, the results definitely showed low blood sugar. Can you imagine how I felt, I had done all this reading and studying and practicing what the books said and felt much better and went to get a glucose tolerance test by doctor "A" only to be referred to doctor "B" when the results indicated something was wrong. And now here was this clown, doctor "B," telling me I suffered from the state of depression and giving me medication for depression.

Nevertheless, being the product of this culture, I still went along with him for a month or so. At first the medication made me feel better. But, as usual, it didn't last which was so typical with me and most medication. My only reason for continuing with him for a month or so was because I was naive enough to believe he might eventually acknowledge I had low blood sugar, but this never happened. At that stage in my life I was still hooked on the belief that I needed the blessings of the medical camp. I am no longer at that point. Are you?

We kept plugging away, reading everything we could about low blood sugar. One thing that kept coming up was the importance of exercise. Jogging was the fad at the time and I tried it every morning but it gave me so much pain that I stopped. Next I tried biking, but that also was too painful so I gave up on exercise. It wasn't until later that I discovered that brisk walking is one of the best exercises you can do—even though it isn't very glamorous. Had I known this at the time I would have walked rather than surrendering and not doing any exercise because of the pain—Oh the hells of low blood sugar.

Then we decided we would be a little unorthodox for a change and I went to a Naturopathic doctor in West Palm Beach. I told him I had low blood sugar and the reason I was coming to him was for information on minerals and vitamins. What a Charlatan he turned out to be, he charged me $90 for about one ounce of fluid he called his "secret formula." My wife would give me injections of this along with the vitamin B_{12} injections. The B_{12} I agree I probably needed but he wouldn't say what was in his own formula. Also he wouldn't tell me where we were headed for as a diet or anything else from one visit to the next. I went to him for a few months which involved about seven visits in all. I kept asking him specific questions and he kept putting me off. I even took my wife with me and that didn't help. So many of these "professionals" are such actors and have the advantage over you when being in such desperate need that they are able to control you.

Now I wonder, "How in the heck did I ever fall into the clutches of that creep?" But when you are suffering, you are constantly groping for that next little something that is going to help you out of the maze. And like most people in this culture I was raised with the idea of seeking authority when needing help with a problem. Until this time I just wasn't willing to be satisfied with the authority of the books alone. Now I am, but it took a long time (seven years) to get here. Also in most of the books it is suggested that you should see a medical person for guidance with low blood sugar. I agree, but it's hard to find one who is willing, able and interested enough.

For the next few months I contented myself with the progress I was able to make due to the books. At this point I saw doctors as being of no benefit to me. Then on one hot, humid and sunny Florida day I decided to work on repairing my dock at the back of our property. Wheeeee—did I do myself in! Normally I do not sweat very much, but that day the sweat literally poured out of me while I worked myself to complete exhaustion. In effect I broke two major principles of maintaining my blood sugar. One is, never do excessive physical work in the heat and another is never work until exhausted. I thought I was about to die, I could barely move, I hurt all over and my eyes hurt severely just with a light being turned on in a room.

So, back to a doctor I went, this time to a G.P. who had treated my son for an earache. In many respects he is one of the few doctors who admitted he only knew enough about low blood sugar to put on his thumb nail. Since I was in such a dire condition he agreed to admit me to the hospital for a complete check up, including another glucose tolerance test and a consultation with an endocrinologist. The results of the GTT again showed low blood sugar and the endocrinologist only told me to continue following the diet suggested in the books.

The couple of times he visited me in my room he kept looking at his watch as if he had somewhere important to go. It really makes a patient feel as if he is in the way and unimportant when his doctor keeps checking his watch. Trying to communicate with him was near impossible. Don't you get to love them?

Finally realizing that we were not going to receive any supportive, reliable services and information from the medical camp, my wife and I decided to dig our oars in deeper and become masters of our own fate.

We began to evaluate and analyze what was happening to me, what with feeling great at times and then sliding way down into the pits other times. Upon taking a close look I realized that I would practice what the books said until I felt improvement and then I would overdo activities and/or work I had't been able to do until feeling better. Also I would begin eating things I shouldn't.

These two errors, I realize now, are common to improving hypoglycemic sufferers. It's almost as if we are bent on destroying the very improvement that we have worked so very hard to gain. Hypoglycemia in itself is not a killer, but it sure makes you suffer. I then decided I would have to pace myself and build brick houses rather than the straw and stick houses that I had been building if I wanted to make good stable progress.

In time I had solved my problem to a large extent which represented about a 70% improvement. However I just couldn't seem to get a handle on 100% at any time with the exception of two short occasions, when I felt like a 1,000,000%. I had never felt like that before. The way I felt was almost mystical, the real Ed Krimmel had come forward even if only for a short time. I wish I could give you a more concise word picture of just how I felt those couple of times. However, as you know, words aren't always able to describe our feelings clearly. But I can tell you I felt completely free of all internal and external forces. It wasn't as if I was feeling all positive, I simply felt like a total force unto myself. I didn't have to expend any energy for this feeling—it was just there. Surrounding me and abounding me. It was just pouring!

I'll let you in on a secret about this feeling—during the time span in which I got the two 1,000,000 percenters I had been following the Food Ethic of the low blood sugar program 100% day in and day out for several months. Also, it was at the time of year when the heat wasn't severe.

I felt that the heat (and the books agreed) of Florida was not the best climate for me. Since it wasn't air pollution that was my problem maybe we should move back to Pennsylvania, our native state. In addition it would be beneficial for our son to be around our relatives and old friends. We moved! So what else was new!

Once back in the Philadelphia, Pennsylvania area (February 1978) I decided to reach out for the other 30% of improvement, this required a more concerted application of all the tools we had studied about in the various books. This included not only diet, but taking the required supplements, exercise and proper amount of rest.

To qualify what I mean by the 70–30% relationship let me just give you a brief overview of where I was at this point.

Symptoms	% of improvement
Headaches	100
Sensitivity to light	95
Tender eyes	95
Cold hands and feet	95
Shortness of breath	70
Tiredness	50
Temper tantrums	95
Irritability	85
Sensitivity to noise	70

Symptoms	*% of improvement*
Anxiety	50
Loss of peripheral vision	95
Knee pains	100
Sleeping difficulties	80
Constant worrying	50
Nightmares	50
Drowsiness	60
Indigestion	80
Forgetfulness	60
Muscle pains	90
Indecisiveness	60
Lack of concentration	50
Phobias-fears	80
Paranoid tendencies	80
Suicide thoughts	99
Bad breath	95

As you can see, a very large boulder of suffering had been lifted from my body and mind. You would have thought that I would have been able to content myself with my improvement, but that was not the case. I felt that somewhere and somehow I could gain a very large part of the additional 30%. Even though most of the physical pain had subsided and mentally I felt super, I felt physically flat. The desire was there, my mind and spirit were willing but I just didn't seem to have a constant energy source on a continuous basis. Sometimes I would get spurts of energy but it wouldn't hold and it wasn't dependable.

Now, I didn't know what to do. Here I was feeling so much better, should I keep trying to get a higher and more dependable level of improvement or leave well enough alone? Try to imagine my frustration, it was 1978 and for the first time after eight long years I started to feel I was in control of my own personal well-being. At what point should I content myself and strike a bargain with fate and low blood sugar for what it is and get on with the other dimensions of my life which had been long neglected and in ill repair. What would you do at this point? Well?

Seventy percent just wasn't enough for me. My wife and I started a campaign to gain the other thirty percent—or as much of it as possible. We decided the best first step would be to go to an endocrinologist on our own since he should know the most about hypoglycemia. You might wonder why we would still be willing to put some trust in a medical doctor. We wonder that ourselves. However, it is very important to maintain hope and we keep hoping that we will find a physician who relates to low blood sugar and its many ramifications.

For the first time we found a doctor who seemed to actually listen to me. He sat there and categorically listed (on paper) what I said. He picked up on things that had never been considered significant by any physician over the years. He thought I might have adrenal insufficiency because of my low blood pressure of 96/70 and the fact that I kept a tan so long. (For some reason the skin pigmentation is darkened when one has adrenal insufficiency). He put me into the hospital for a week where a complete work up was done, including another GTT, which again indicated low blood sugar. By the fourth hour of the test I was really feeling terrible with sweating, severe jumpy feelings and faintness. Later I learned my blood sugar was at 47 mg at the fourth hour which is excessively low. Other tests indicated that I had partial adrenal insufficiency. Later I discovered, after more reading, that adrenal insufficiency and low blood sugar often go hand in hand. I was put on prednisone and sudafed for the adrenal insufficiency and told to continue my diet. The medications did give me that extra lift of 5–10% but as time went on the sudafed was increased to such a point that I was told to check my blood pressure often because sudafed can cause an unhealthy rise in blood pressure. Also prednisone is a medication which should be taken with great caution because of its potential side effects.

Well now—I guess the average person would just sit back, put his feet up and say, ain't this sweet and go right along with the situation, but not me. At this point my big fear was that I might find myself, after 8 years of suffering and searching to find out what was wrong with me, in a worse situation than ever, what with having to check my blood pressure regularly and the threat of prednisone's side effects looming in the shadows. Now I found myself on a different type of ice cube and banana peel. I knew too often the pills of medicine bear no health.

After having been on these medications for at least six months, I decided to see a doctor in the area who was supposedly nutritionally oriented. My thought was that I might have a chance of getting closer to capturing as much of the 30% as possible by using vitamins and mineral supplements instead of medications. On my first visit to this physician he did blood work, stool analysis and hair analysis. He also began decreasing the prednisone and sudafed which he felt were doing more harm than good. By my next visit he had received the results of the various tests and could start me on appropriate vitamin and mineral supplements. I also began receiving vitamin B_{12} injections and taking adrenal extract in place of the prednisone and sudafed.

Having chosen to take this alternate course I had to bear in mind that the supplements would lead to a long term gradual improvement in contrast to the quick fix of the medications. I continued seeing this physician for approximately five months and noticed a gradual additional increase in my well-being. One extremely conspicuous improvement occurred which pertained to something I haven't mentioned before, because at the time I didn't think it was related to my body chemistry. Since 1968 my finger and toe nails had gradually been deteriorating to the point where most of them were completely missing only to be replaced by a thick, hard, callous like substance. I had been told it was due to psoriasis and no medication was ever helpful. Imagine my surprise when after 9–10 months of taking the supplements my nails not only stopped deteriorating but began to regenerate. As of this writing I have all finger nails and toenails.

My reasons for not continuing to see the physician who started me on supplements are that he really didn't have any in-depth understanding of low blood sugar and the suffering it causes. He knew all the "buzz words" to use but when I questioned him in-depth about certain concepts he became defensive and wasn't able to give adequate answers. Something else that alarmed me about him occurred on one of my last visits to his office when he was administering a six hour glucose tolerance test to a woman. This woman was sitting in the waiting room while having the test and was having severe reactions to the test such as faintness, sweating, vision difficulties and trembling. Her husband didn't know what to do and was not aware that these were some of the side effects of the test. I helped him get her from the chair to a sofa where she could lie down and then told the receptionist to get the doctor. In a short time the doctor appeared from his inner office and merely looked at her very superficially and returned to his office after making some vague comments to the woman and her husband. He didn't give them any insight into what was happening or why. I couldn't believe what I was witnessing. Here was a human being suffering some very severe reactions from the test and not being given any support or comfort—just ignored in that typical, ever so popular fashion known to the medical vocation. How did they ever learn to "treat" humans in such an offhanded style?

Another reason I lost faith in this doctor and stopped going to him was because he had me coming to him on a biweekly basis for vitamin B_{12} injections. Since my wife is a nurse, I asked him to give me a prescription for the B_{12} and my wife would give me the injections. This would save me time and money. He would not go along with the idea and couldn't give me any good reason for not doing so.

I would estimate that I improved another 10% by taking the supplements. This left me with 20% more to go. I decided (the books kept telling me too) that I must begin a conscientious exercise program of one kind or another. Since it was winter, my wife and I started with a very small amount of gentle calisthenics. Gradually I was able to increase the calisthenics and in addition began taking brisk walks daily. By late Spring we began playing noncompetitive, fun tennis every morning and continued with the brisk walks. Sometimes we include bike riding and swimming. These activities have added an additional 10%, bringing me now up to 90% improvement. I love it, I love it.

My general feelngs are, I could gain this last 10% by somehow being able to get more involved working to help other people with low blood sugar problems. During the times when I'm totally engrossed with other low blood sugar sufferers, I find my time is spent with a sense of accomplishment and fulfillment. Due to my basic personality traits, accomplishment and fulfillment are vital to my overall feeling of wellness, monetary gain does not have top priority. Sometimes I think it is good not to have monetary gains as my top priority. The wonderful feelings we have enjoyed over these years in helping many individuals are priceless.

As of this writing I am in great shape and feel more together than ever before. I am still looking for a knowledgeable, interested, nutritionally oriented doctor. In some respects I do not need a physician but from a practical standpoint it would be nice to have a doctor in whom I have confidence.

I would like to express a special "Thank You" to my wife for being the wonderful human being she is—without her help I couldn't have made the progress or gained the insights I have.

Anyone for a brisk walk?

Ed Krimmel's (author) GTT results:

year	fasting	½ hr	1 hr	2 hr	3 hr	4 hr	5 hr	6 hr
1976	95	124	90	78	88	85	72	70
1977	95	195	194	136	75	85	72	81
1978	86	140	145	118	77	47	76	83

KEY
1976 ....
1977 ------------
1978 ————

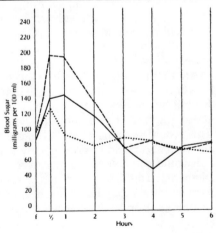

Other Case Histories

Following is a letter and case history received from a fellow low blood sugar victim and sufferer:

Dear Ed and Pat,   April, 1979

I just received your information and want to commend you on compiling some excellent tips for hypoglycemics.

My intention is to include with this letter a case study which I typed up in June 1977. Much has changed since then. As stated, I intend to use this letter as an addendum to the case study.

I have read about 10 to 12 books related to my problem. After having read 6 or so I finally truly grasped the situation.

As a rundown I had about 90% of the symptoms listed including psycho-motor seizures (treated wtih Phenobarbital and Mysolin) and extreme suicidal bouts (treated by a psychiatrist I could not afford). Next to these two, anything else seemed minor and only added to my portrait as a "lazy bitch." I maintained a job but did very poorly—something incongruous to my basic nature and therefore hard to understand. Yes, I lost my husband through it all. But to be where I am now is worth it.

I presently have problems only when I deviate from the diet and/or have extreme stress.

I had no problems with seizures from August, 1975 to January, 1979. I still don't understand what happened. I certainly had been under more stress in the interim time but . . . nevertheless . . . I have about 3 days of seizures each month since then.

I take "mucho" vitamins. For example: 50–75 IU vitamin A, vitamin B complex, 1,000 mg vitamin C, 1,000 IU vitamin E, a multiple vitamin, a multi-mineral, 3–4 papaya tablets, B_6, dolomite (a natural anti-convulsant), 3 desiccated liver, 2 TBS. brewer's yeast in water, and 1 TBS. lecithen each day.

Other than my few problem times I've never felt or looked so good. I'm very busy with my new business and find snacking sometimes a problem but generally am very good. We are now opening store #3 (referring to case study again) and have plans for more.

Sincerely, Anonymous

I am 30-years-old, quite intelligent, very intense in my interpersonal relationships with people, always trying "to please." I was a major in chemistry with aspirations to become a doctor. Due to my mental state at that time in my life it became an impossibility.

I began to have what I would now diagnose as petit mal seizures when I was a senior in high school. The "family doctor" said I was merely high strung and nervous and prescribed Librium. I was in an accelerated academic class at school and my one main fear was that I would have one of these "things" during a timed-test while at school. They seemed to happen when I was in a stressful situation. I went away to college and the seizures continued for about 1 ½ years and gradually faded away. In the meantime, more of my nervousness appeared. I had been, and continued to be, a constant worrier, I would move jerkily, seemingly without coordination. I, in fact, joked quite often about my lack of coordination in relationship to my lack of athletic ability. I was not tuned into my body as well as I am now, so I am not even aware of all that was going on. I had great difficulty maintaining anything but superficial friendships, even though I knew I was a very nice person. I seemed to be crying on the phone to my parents a couple of times a week.

I was graduated from college and began working for a chemical company in Columbus, Ohio. My grades from college were not what I knew I was capable of. I had great difficulty concentrating. Now I wonder how I did some of the things I did with such a difficult major and losing the ability to study.

Later I got a laboratory job with a research firm in Pennsylvania. I had gained weight after returning from Columbus and decided to go on an "Ayds" diet. Daily I smoked a pack of cigarettes, drank several cups of coffee with 3 tsps. of sugar, and ate my "Ayds." I don't believe I was even eating breakfast—never had except for donuts or toast with cinnamon-sugar. I ate one meal a day. I also became engaged that summer to a childhood acquaintance. We had severe religious problems. Interestingly enough, I also began having seizures—much worse this time.

Frank, my fiance, encouraged me to see a neurologist while the people at work encouraged me to see a neuro-psychiatrist. The second sent me on to the first recommendation (expensive advice). The neurologist diagnosed it as Psycho-motor Epilepsy. I was to take 3 Mysoline daily. Frank wanted me to take them, my family didn't. I didn't know what to do. I will always remember the day I took just ½ a tablet. It was like drawing a curtain around me and losing touch with reality. I knew that I was only going to step back deeper and deeper and this was to be my life sentence! That is why I was hesitant at first and later decided to take 1 per day. Over a period of about 2 years I began to take the 3 pills.

I fear that this is becoming too detailed so I am going to attempt to make more generalized statements . . .

I went to a series of doctors. I also got married in the meantime. There was never a period when I felt I was free of the seizures. I would go as much as three months without them and then have a really bad flock of them. All the doctors explained that it was epilepsy but didn't know why. I can remember asking one doctor if there was a possibility that it could be a chemical imbalance—perhaps I was missing a nutrient or element that other people had. He laughed at me and amusedly explained that this was just not possible.

One MD (these were all specialists, of course!) prescribed Dilantin along with my Mysoline. I began to have pain in my teeth and gums soon after that. I was totally unaware that there could be a connection.

I normally tried to "hide my affliction" but for some reason went to a dentist and we discussed the fact that I had the beginning of hyperplasia. He asked what drugs I was taking. The Dilantin was causing it. I called my Neurologist and he said, "Well, you'd better stop taking it" . . . I did.

During this time I began to get the overwhelming urge to commit suicide. I couldn't get in touch with myself at this time and didn't know why this was happening. I decided that I must really be unhappy for this to happen. Most of the time I thought things were okay. I did have a few things that needed to be worked on. I was much too dependent on Frank, in fact I suffocated him. I couldn't make decisions and needed him to guide my every move. I was walking on very shaky ground. The feelings of suicide frightened me so much that I began telling Frank. It was more than he could handle. I think he tried every approach possible.

I had received my Masters degree in Education (40 hours in one year while working full-time) and we were both teaching in Germany—1972–1974.

We returned to the States—Frank was a licensed funeral director—bought an old home to remodel into a funeral home, and proceeded to live happily ever after. Frank was concerned about my having children with my mental state and was also concerned about my passing on the epilepsy to our children. I had a job I hated (living on donuts, coffee still with 3 tsps. of sugar and my faithful pack of cigarettes). I couldn't cope effectively with the remodeling; I began looking like a hag; I didn't realize how much I was letting myself go. I began to feel more often that there was absoutely nothing to live for. Frank became more distraught. I recall one weekend I lay in bed and didn't move for the whole weekend. Frank would occasionally come in and look at me, shake his head and leave and continue to work on the remodeling. I have always had a slight weight problem, varying from 10 to 20 pounds overweight. I was never extremely confident but the lack of confidence seemed to intensify. I didn't want anyone to see me or to see anyone. I must have been horrible to live with. We went to see a marriage counselor and he told me that I needed a psychiatrist. He secretly told Frank that if it were up to him he would admit me to a psychiatric hospital and begin shock treatments immediately. Fortunately Frank couldn't bear to do that.

In the meantime, my father was quite a health enthusiast. My parents were living in Florida at the time. He suggested that I had hypoglycemia. I had never heard of it and neither had Frank. My father told me how to tackle it (according to his reading). I, however, was too far gone to help myself and Frank didn't (admittedly, now) quite believe him. I began going to the psychiatrist recommended by the marriage counselor. I couldn't drive because I had epilepsy, so Frank had to take time out of a busy schedule and drive me every Thursday night. It cost $40 each time! I would go through a series of several mood changes just on the way to the office. The MD seemed intent on dealing with my fantasies and not the real problem. I suggested that (according to my father) it may be hypoglycemia. He replied that very few people have this condition and he intended to have me checked by an internist and he would know. I was checked and he detected nothing by the one blood sample.

I am embarrassed, this is turning into a book.

My marriage with Frank was disintegrating and he encouraged me to visit my parents in Florida for awhile. I did. My father began to encourage me to follow the low blood sugar diet; take vitamins daily, drink 2 to 4 Tbsp. of Brewer's yeast daily, take lecithin, omit sugar in any form from my diet, cease eating white flour—and the result was miraculous! I also quit smoking. I began exercising on the beach and used the spa. When I returned home everyone noticed the dramatic change, except Frank. Things had just gone too far. I, nevertheless, had now begun to feel good enough that I didn't let that stop my progress. I was taking an interest in my appearance again too. I still had a few really bad times. I returned in September, 1976. I began to launch into getting ready for Christmas and made all of my Christmas gifts, baked, etc. Even with the bad times, the difference in my lifestyle remained.

In January, 1977 I received what I thought was the final blow. Frank told me he just didn't love me anymore. I, of course, had to leave. He couldn't leave a budding business. That is said a little sarcastically, but it really was the only logical solution at the time. I went to Philadelphia and stayed with the only person I knew there until I got a secretarial job. I drank too much for about 3 months. It seemed the only way I could cope. The ironic thing is that I continued to take my vitamins! After getting settled I found a doctor specializing in hypoglycemia. I at last had a Glucose Tolerance Test. I knew when I was taking the test and lying on the table unable to move that something was wrong. The results proved to be hypoglycemia. I am enclosing the results. The doctor asked me to take a further test, to ingest cortisone and have a 2 hour GTT. He said I was a pre-diabetic. I accepted that diagnosis and he wanted me to take Meltrol or DBI (you may have heard of this drug being taken off the market because of fatal side reactions). I took it but had a recurrence of severe emotional disturbances—noticeable by the people at work. I called the doctor, crying hysterically, and tried to tell him what I thought had happened. He said to go off of it. Fortunately, my body reacted this way.

I failed to tell you that I was placed on 3 Mysoline and 3 Phenolbarbitols in 1974 and since the trip to Florida had had no seizures, among all the other good things. I began to very gradually go off of all six pills. By December 31, 1976 I had taken my last one!!! What a great day. The curtain was lifted.

There are still a few things I am working on. I have eliminated every possible vice. I was drinking Sanka and tea, and still having periods when I just could not cope with my everyday problems and suicide was the only answer. I have not located a doctor in my area of Florida to monitor the Hypoglycemia yet so I called one in Fort Lauderdale. She suggested that maybe the tea was causing this problem. I haven't had tea or Sanka for 10 days now. I must admit that hasn't happened again. Only time will tell. I have run out of things to eliminate. I am eating every 2 hours and following my diet strictly. I actually have times when I feel *"really good." You don't know how thankful I am.*

Oh, a further addition to my life. I am planning to go into business with my mother and sister selling frozen yogurt (I know I can't eat the product) with fresh fruit and dry toppings.

At least I have a bright future. Think of all the people barely making it through life and having a similar problem.

GLUCOSE TOLERANCE TEST RESULTS

fasting	½ hr	1 hr	2 hr	3 hr	4 hr	5 hr	6 hr
65	65	80	35	70	50	60	65

Paul—A 5-year-old, medically diagnosed as having low blood sugar after having a series of blackouts, leg pains, tiredness and other symptoms. A medical doctor told his parents to give him a snack before going to bed and that eventually he would outgrow the problem and there was no need to stop him from eating sugar and put him on a special diet. The parents of this child preferred listening 100% to the medical camp even to the extent that they would not read books or try anything other than what the formal medical camp recommended.

Meanwhile, you have a child who is blacking out, having leg pains, etc., etc., etc. What an interesting form of child abuse. A thought to ponder is, if the child had been diagnosed as having high blood sugar (diabetes) would they have accepted the idea that he would eventually outgrow the condition. The simple facts are that the person diagnosed with high blood sugar—diabetes—does not outgrow it, it must be treated either with diet or medication and diet. Why then should these parents, or the doctor, readily accept the idea that a person will outgrow low blood sugar—hypoglycemia?

The mother appeared to be interested in information, but when we spoke to the father he asked in a very sarcastic tone: "What are you on, a crusade or something?" Unfortunately, we were unable to give any aid other than giving the mother some pertinent printed information.

Father M.—A 40-year-old parish priest. Eight years ago Father M. was diagnosed as having hypoglycemia. The only information given to him by his doctor at that time was to drink orange juice when he didn't feel right. Father M. continued to suffer the many ramifications of hypoglycemia— (awakening 5 to 6 times a night, waking up very tired and as if he had been beaten during the night, feeling as if he weighed a ton when getting out of bed, and suffering blackouts, anxiety, momentary memory difficulties, etc., etc., etc.

Within 3 days after our initial in depth discussion and recommendations, Father M. was sleeping all night and had 50% improvement of his condition on awakening. Within two months he was 75 to 90% improved in the various areas mentioned above. He was asked by his family and friends what he had done to gain back his old happy disposition and to lose weight.

Over the past several years he had had great difficulty in maintaining his work load as a parish priest, but now he is able to handle it with very little difficulty.

Father M. is a classic example of a person suffering with a low blood sugar problem who had never been given adequate information and support to sufficiently handle the problem. However, now he has the information to gain insight into his low blood sugar situation. Now Father M. can relate to any progress or setbacks he may experience from day to day.

Ron—A 32-year-old school teacher, husband and father of a small son. Ron was diagnosed as a hypoglycemic 7 years ago. His doctor made one specific statement with no supportive information: "Eat plenty of protein and avoid sweets." Ron followed this general diet for a short period of time and got very favorable results. For 3 classic reasons Ron did not continue on this general diet and therefore his progress stopped.

1. There was no in depth explanation of low blood sugar given to him, therefore he did not understand why following the diet was so important and made him feel so much better.
2. Ron was not told to avoid all white flour products, stimulants (caffeine, tobacco and alcohol), and highly concentrated carbohydrate foods.
3. There was a total lack of supportive personal interest, which is found to be vital to people with low blood sugar. (See Pilot-Co-pilot section.)

Ron's primary complaints were irritabiltiy, argumentativeness, depression, prevailing fatigue, craving for sweets (ate at least one 1-pound Hershey bar daily), unsocial behavior etc., etc. He was also extremely concerned and upset about the severity with which he was disciplining his 4-year-old son. So much so that he would often have tremendous feelings of remorse and guilt and cry by his son's bed while the child was asleep.

At the time of our initial contact with Ron he had his house for sale, was contemplating divorce and quitting his job. Within a month of instruction and encouragement to Ron and his wife, he was making a complete turnabout. He decided to keep his wife, home and job and is now living very happily. He no longer has reason to have remorse or guilt about the way he treats his son.

The last time we spoke to Ron, he was following the program very conscientiously and eagerly anticipating the arrival of another child.

Bob—A 28-year-old, bright, enthusiastic real estate agent. He has never felt it necessary to have a glucose tolerance test because of the great success he has had in feeling so much better by faithfully following the Krimmel Program. Bob's attitude and question is; the test isn't going to make me feel any better but the program does, so why do I need the test?

True, and a good point. However we have asked Bob to talk it over with an Endocrinologist about how he used to feel and how he feels now. Also to ask the doctor to put him in the hospital to do a thorough body chemistry work-up.

When we first met Bob, his life seemed to have been shredded into pieces of confetti. In starting to work with him one of the first things we had to do was to try to help him put the pieces into some sort of order and at the same time start on the program. Apparently the price Bob was paying in pain and frustration was very obvious to him because he has been one of the most pleasurable individuals to work with. From day one he has always been anxious, and sometimes impatient, to reach out for that next rung of improvement. Too often it is we who have to encourage the person to reach out for the next rung on the ladder, but with Bob it has always been his initiative. Another nice part about Bob is that he is able to remember clearly how he used to feel and is easily able to see how much progress he has made. Most individuals tend to forget how they used to feel once they have made significant progress on the program.

Here are a few of Bob's complaints:

Anxiety	Excessive nervous laughter
Motor mouth (can't stop talking)	Impatience
Sleep difficulties	Mood swings
Headaches	Deterioration of self-esteem
Short concentration span	Sensitivity to light (wore sunglasses all
Confusion	day)

As long as Bob follows the program he can enjoy conspicuous and significant benefits. Being young and a social person, one of his biggest problems is when he is socializing. Invariably after having a couple of beers he pays the price for the next day or two. We always tell him, if you want to play, you've got to pay, that's the harsh reality of it.

Before we met Bob he was already using vitamins and minerals. Within a few months Bob has made tremendous inroads in piecing his life together, so much so, that he can now reach out to other members of his family. He has had a major improvement in his career and is now more able to adopt a greater quantity of responsibility and degree of professionalism. There is only one thing wrong with Bob, he won't stop thanking us, this is the price we have had to pay. Bob has been a pleasure to help.

Hank—A 45-year-old entrepreneur, diagnosed as having low blood sugar. Hank's first indication of low blood sugar came quite by accident. I was telling him about my own problems with low blood sugar and the price I had paid because of it. While talking to him I noticed a change in his expression. His eyes started to shine and he got a wry smile, which caused me to ask; "Do you get feelings like these?"

To make a long story short, Hank had the glucose tolerance test and was diagnosed as having low blood sugar. His doctor told him to drink Coke when he felt tired or weak and gave him a "mickey mouse" diet. So much for doctors and Disneyland. Hank had been given unreliable information and no support.

We supplied Hank with pertinent information and an extended period of supportive help, including a week's supply of snack parcels. Unfortunately, we are too far out of reach on a regular basis and he needs someone close to be totally supportive. In our opinion, until he sees the light and learns to take care of himself, or gets someone filling this role, he will remain in the clouds, paying the price for his blood sugar not being stabilized.

We are happy to report that he has stopped drinking Cokes and was surprised by the positive improvements, one being less anxiety.

His primary need is to have someone make up food parcels everyday and to have someone insist he eats regularly.

Then he should pursue activities for the purpose of having fun, not excitement, or relaxation or because they're interesting. But fun, fun, fun, because fun and laughter are very beneficial tonics.

Amusement parks and sporting events are exciting and can be forms of fun. But the dimension of fun we are talking about is fun associated with laughter and a feeling of release. A few activities which give us a great amount of fun, laughter and release are unorganized softball games, unorganized volleyball games, sledding and humorous plays and movies.

The number one priority of the LBS sufferer must be his individual health and personal well-being. Hank has yet to pay adequate attention to this Number-One priority. It's not as if he doesn't get any pain. But so far, it seems he would rather have the pain and live off his glands than the proper food, rest, exercise and fun.

Here is a brief list of his symptoms:

Severe headaches	Depression
Upset stomach	Exhaustion
Short concentration span	Irritability
Over magnification of problems	Mood swings
Excessive worrying	Indecisiveness

Hank would hardly be suspected of having LBS. Here is a gentleman who has a very high success curve running five businesses, seems to have a successful and happy family life and is an avid skier and tennis player. I personally don't know how he ever does it. He is one of the biggest contradictions of LBS sufferers I know. Most LBS sufferers have a fragmented lifestyle. The best I can say is that Hank has been very successful at living off his glands and has been a mastermind at planning. Just think what he could achieve with his LBS regulated.

Beneath Hank's layers of success lives a full blossomed Low Blood Sugar victim. He has a vast collection of severe symptoms and is a victim of one of the most harsh and common LBS problems—getting his priorities in order.

Susan—A 22-year-old secretary. She was diagnosed as having low blood sugar and told by her physician to go and find out about it on her own, since he didn't know that much about it.

This physician deserves special acknowledgment for his straight-fowardness and honesty in admitting his lack of information on LBS.

Susan originally went to her doctor because she had blacked out a few times. Other symptoms were waking up tired, nervousness, cold hands and feet, headaches, fatigue and stuttering.

She is a young, exciting person who is anxious to be on the move and doing exciting things even though she suffers some severe consequences such as blacking out occasionally. In reality, Susan doesn't have to slow down but she must alter some of her habits—order seltzer water with lemon rather than alcohol, herb tea rather than regular tea or coffee (or carry herb tea with her).

While on vacation Susan blacked out on the beach. She was carried to the shade where she shortly regained consciousness. When she reported this to her doctor he said it was due to the sun. I asked her if the sun was all that severe and how many other people passed out. She said the sun was not severe and no one else of the hundreds on the beach passed out. That being the case, I told her it was most likely due to her LBS. The sun can cause stress, particularly since she had not eaten for an extended period of time. It is very important for a LBS victim to take food to the beach and to sit under a beach umbrella since heat from the sun can cause excessive stress on a LBS sufferer.

Susan's progress has been in direct proportion to the degree she follows our program.

Sarah—A 22-year-old cafe waitress was never formally diagnosed as having low blood sugar. Sarah became very interested in LBS when we were working with her mother, who had been diagnosed several years earlier as having LBS.

Sarah already knew that certain things, such as sugar and alcohol, made her feel terrible. She also had sleeping problems—waking up 6 to 7 times during the night and then being exhausted in the morning. Therefore, she could not hold a daytime job because she wasn't able to get up on time. In addition, she would be very grumpy in the morning. Who wouldn't be? Headaches occurred frequently.

Shortly after talking with us and reading some information we gave her she began following our advice. Her symptoms started to erode and a new person and lifestyle began to emerge. Sarah had always wanted to have a 9 to 5 job so her evenings would be free for socializing. Since she was now able to sleep through the night and get up in the morning refreshed and cheerful (providing she ate immediately before going to bed), she changed her job and became a 9 to 5 secretary.

Mary—A 35-year-old legal secretary, divorced and living with her 13-year-old son. She complained of sleeping problems, headaches, depression, super tiredness, muscle aches, forgetfulness, sensitivity to bright lights and noises, craving for sweets and junk food, indecisiveness, falling and stumbling, itchy skin, excessive desire for club soda (40 oz. a day), heart palpitations, sweating and hot flashes. Her doctor prescribed thyroid medication and tranquilizers daily and a diuretic once every 2 weeks. These medications did not help.

After work, Mary usually had 4 to 5 drinks before going home and then had difficulty staying awake on the way home. Her whole life was a nightmare.

We supplied Mary with information along with many hours of counseling. Although Mary had all these problems on a regular basis, all she wanted help with was getting a good night's sleep. For the past 4 to 5 years she had only been getting 2 to 3 hours sleep nightly.

Here is what we suggested to her:

- Have no stimulants after 8 p.m. (caffeine, nicotine, alcohol).
- Go to bed every night at the same time, approximately 11:30 p.m.
- Eat either a hard boiled egg or 6 ounces of plain yogurt immediately before getting into bed.
- Keep yogurt at the bedside and eat some in the event you wake up during the night.

By the end of one week, Mary was sleeping through the night.

Mary felt she needed a support group in order to follow the complete program. To date we have not offered this because the individuals we have worked with have been scattered over too large an area.

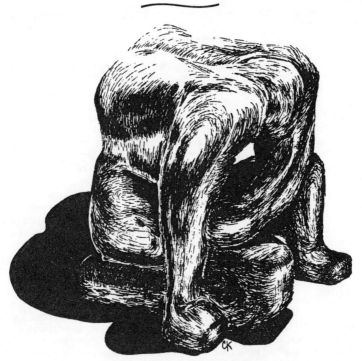

Thought in Black and White

Sculpture—Albert E. Krimmel
Pen & Ink—Charles A. Krimmel

Chapter 2

WHAT IS HYPOGLYCEMIA, LOW BLOOD SUGAR?

Hypoglycemia is the formal name for low blood sugar (LBS). Hypo is the Greek word for below and glycemia means sugar or glucose in the blood. Low blood sugar is a condition where the amount of glucose (sugar) in the blood is below the amount needed for the body to function properly.

WHAT IS BLOOD SUGAR?

Blood sugar is the sugar in your blood. The sugar in your blood is glucose. The sugar in your sugar bowl is sucrose which is comprised of two sugars, glucose and fructose.

The glucose in your blood is measured by how many milligrams (mg) (1 mg is equal to .0003 oz.) of glucose is in 100 cubic centimeters (cc) (approximately 3 ⅓ oz.) of your blood.

Normal blood sugar is usually considered to be 80–120 mg of glucose per 100 cc of blood. Abnormal blood sugar is usually considered anything above 160 mg or below 65 mg.

Anyone with blood sugar above 160 mg is suspected of being diabetic (*hyper*glycemia). Anyone with blood sugar below 65 mg is suspect of having low blood sugar (*hypo*glycemia). However, the real qualifier is how you feel and what symptoms you are experiencing, not the numbers.

WHY DO WE NEED GLUCOSE?

Glucose is the fuel the body burns for energy and heat. This fuel is necessary for your body to run properly, just as your car needs fuel (gas) to run. Glucose is used by every cell in your body for energy and heat. Your brain and the retina of your eye use only glucose for fuel, though your other cells are able to use fats or amino acids (from proteins) if necessary.

Most of your cells store glucose in the form of glycogen and when glucose is needed the cells convert glycogen to glucose. The central nervous system—the key part of which is the brain—does not store glucose and therefore is the first area to be affected by low blood sugar.

Since the brain doesn't store glucose it is totally dependent on the amount of glucose that is in the blood stream. When the glucose in the blood is low the brain doesn't receive enough energy and therefore is unable to function efficiently and is affected before any other part of your body. Just think about that for a while and let its significance burn deep into your mind.

FROM WHERE DO WE GET GLUCOSE?

Our best source of glucose is carbohydrate foods. Carbohydrates are starches and sugars. Foods rich in carbohydrates are grains, seeds, beans, vegetables and fruits. Unrefined (nonprocessed) carbohydrates are made up of long-chain molecules and during digestion are *slowly* broken down into smaller molecules of glucose. Refined (processed) carbohydrates (white flour and sugar products, etc.) are made up of short-chain molecules and are broken down into glucose much *faster* during digestion.

Amino acids from proteins and glycerol from fats can be converted by the cells to glucose if the need arises.

PHYSIOLOGY OF LOW BLOOD SUGAR

Physiology is the study of the functions of cells, tissues, and organs of the human body. Following is a brief overview of the physiology of low blood sugar.

Digestion

The digestive system is comprised of the mouth, salivary glands, esophagus, stomach, small and large intestines, pancreas, liver and gall bladder. This system performs various chemical, thermal and mechanical actions to break down the food you eat.

The chemical makeup of a food determines how long it remains in the stomach. Carbohydrates remain only a few hours, protein a little longer and fatty food may remain many hours.

The salivary glands secrete ptyalin, an enzyme which begins to break down carbohydrates while you are chewing. Gastric juices continue to digest the food in your stomach and the digestion is completed in the small intestine by digestive juices secreted by the pancreas and gall bladder. These digestive juices break down food into molecules that are small enough to be absorbed through the intestinal wall into the blood stream (see Fig. 1).

Absorption

These molecules are absorbed through the intestinal wall in the form of nutrients; glucose from carbohydrates, amino acids from pro-

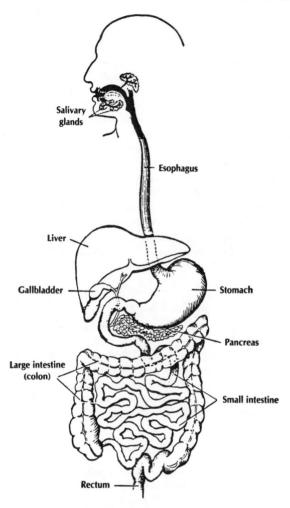

Fig. 1 Digestive System.

teins, and fatty acids and glycerol from fats. The glucose, amino acids and some fatty acids and glycerol go through the intestinal wall into the blood stream of the portal vein. The portal vein transports the nutrients and blood to the liver.

Glucose Transportation

When the nutrients reach the liver some are absorbed to be used by the liver itself, some are stored for later use and the balance are released into the blood stream and carried to the cells of the body that need them. For example, when the nutrient glucose enters the liver, some of it is converted to glycogen and stored, some is used immediately by the liver cells and the rest is carried by the blood stream to cells that need it for heat and/or energy.

In order for glucose to enter a cell, insulin, which comes from the pancreas, must be present in the blood stream. If too much insulin is present then too much glucose enters the cells and the glucose in the blood stream falls too low and you have low blood sugar, hypoglycemia. If on the other hand, there is no insulin or too little insulin being sent to the blood stream by the pancreas, then the glucose is not able to enter the cells, leaving too much glucose in the blood stream and you have diabetes, hyperglycemia. This is an overly simplified explanation but it gives a basic picture of what seems to be the underlying potential cause of low blood sugar and diabetes (hypoglycemia and hyperglycemia) which are both related to the inadequate regulation of glucose possibly caused by too much or too little insulin being released by the pancreas or the insulin not being used correctly.

Possible Causes of Low Blood Sugar

Whatever the cause, it seems obvious that some people's body chemistry cannot handle sugar, fruits, starchy foods, alcohol and/or stimulants (caffeine, nicotine etc). These substances cause a variety of symptoms and suffering for some people. At the present there is no known definite cause of low blood sugar.

There may be many causes for improper sugar metabolism and regulation, some of which may be:

- Too much insulin being released
- Under or over active adrenal glands
- Liver disorder
- Excessive amounts of refined carbohydrates in diet
- Disorders of pituitary or thyroid glands
- Tumor of pancreas
- Trauma

Most of the regulation of the amount of glucose in the blood is controlled by the liver, pancreas, adrenal glands, thyroid gland, pituitary gland and the brain. If your blood sugar goes too low, the brain sends a signal via the pituitary and thyroid glands to the adrenal glands which release adrenalin that goes to the liver and signals the liver to convert stored glycogen to glucose. The glucose is sent into the blood stream and carried to the cells of the body that require it and the pancreas releases insulin so the glucose can be utilized by the cells. Thus, you can see how the improper functioning of one or more glands can disrupt sugar metabolism (see Fig. 2).

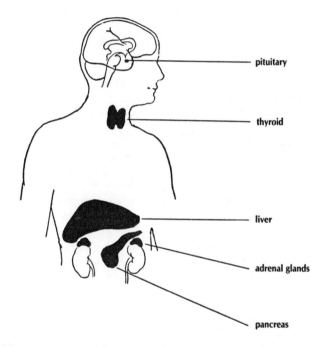

Pituitary–secretes growth hormone which influences food metabolism. Releases hormones which increase activity of adrenal cortex and thyroid gland.

Thyroid–produces hormones controlling metabolic rate of body.

Liver–extracts, processes and stores nutrients. Converts glucose to glycogen for storage and converts it back to glucose when needed.

Adrenals–produce cortisol and aldosterone in response to ACTH from pituitary. Cortisol affects glucose, amino acid and fat metabolism. Also secretes adrenaline which stimulates liver to put out glucose when needed.

Pancreas–produces insulin which enables glucose to enter and be used by the cells, also reduces glucose production in liver.

Fig. 2.   Organs That Help to Regulate Blood Sugar.

There are two broad classifications of LBS:

1. Organic—very rare form of LBS. Symptoms are caused by a gland, (pancreas, liver, adrenal or pituitary, etc.) having a defect or tumor which can be medically isolated and demonstrated. Once the problem is corrected, the symptoms leave.
2. Functional—something in your body chemistry is not functioning properly. The most common theory is that symptoms are caused by an over active/over sensitive pancreas which releases too much insulin. This theory is based on the idea that LBS is the opposite of diabetes where the pancreas is under active/under sensitive and releases too little or no insulin. Functional LBS has two divisions:
   Reactive—LBS symptoms occur shortly after eating certain foods. Your body chemistry reacts negatively to those foods.
   Fasting—LBS symptoms occur as a result of not eating for an extended period of time.

Why Symptoms Occur

It is when your blood sugar is too low that your symptoms occur because certain areas of the body are not receiving enough energy from glucose to function properly. Usually the first areas to be affected when your glucose is low are your central nervous system and eyes because they use only glucose for energy. This is why it is common for low blood sugar individuals to have irritability, nervousness, anxiety, headaches, vertigo, drowsiness, visual disturbances, forgetfulness, insomnia, faintness, exhaustion, etc. So the next time you feel like your "plug is being pulled out" think low blood sugar and eat some appropriate food. (See chapter 4.)

HOW SERIOUS IS LOW BLOOD SUGAR?

"How serious is low blood sugar?" We think low blood sugar is the most dangerous condition in the U.S. today. Its seriousness ranges from a headache to suicide. Here is a condition that has no prejudice, it simply doesn't care what color you are, what nationality you are, what religion you are or what your income is or anything else about you. It can disable you no matter what.

The numbers are staggering, estimates of the number of people in the U.S. with low blood sugar tendencies range from 50 million to 75 million. Once you learn enough about the subject and start watching closely and listening to people around you, you'll begin to think that everyone has it. At this point we advise you to be prudent in relating to others about low blood sugar, it can be dangerous to your social relationships. If you feel you must help someone, suggest some books for the person to read.

If not diagnosed or not maintained after diagnosis, the following are some common problems of low blood sugar sufferers.

Domestic Problems

Because of the uneven emotional plane of the low blood sugar person, the domestic setting can become very explosive and lead to:

- Wife—husband abuse
- Child abuse
- Employment difficulties (late, argumentive, low productivity, etc.)
- Divorce or separation

Children's Difficulties

Learning difficulties—The brain requires a constant supply of energy from glucose in order to function properly. How can a child's brain be expected to receive and process information correctly and comfortably if it is not receiving an adequate and constant supply of energy from glucose?

Behavior problems at home and school—Poor concentration and attention span, irritability, hostility, low self-esteem, etc. can very often be attributed to low blood sugar.

Juvenile delinquency and crime—There have been studies in youth centers that show that a majority of these youths have low blood sugar. These studies show a strong relationship between aggressive criminal activity and a low quality diet. In Pitkin County, Colorado, prisoners that went on a diet free of white flour, sugar, and coffee had no trouble with the law after their release. In Dougherty County, Georgia, every juvenile offender gets a biochemical test and is given nutritional supplements. Dougherty County enjoys the lowest juvenile crime rate in the nation. In Cuyahoga Falls, Ohio, 600 criminals were given nutritional education and a diet high in whole grains and fresh fruits and vegetables, 89% of them did not have a repeat crime. Some other jails and detention centers have removed white flour, sugar, and junk foods from the environment, the results have been improved relations between everyone with inmates taking an interest in themselves and their well-being. When these individuals follow the "junk free" diet after leaving the institutions their rate of returning to crime is much less than those who continue on the typical junk food diet. A low blood sugar individual usually has a very low boiling point when his sugar is low, therefore when unregulated, it is very easy for him to lose his temper and get into fights which can and often do lead to more serious situations.

Alcohol and Drug Abuse

Studies reveal that the majority of alcoholics and drug addicts have low blood sugar. If you ever attend an AA meeting, you will be amazed at the amount of coffee, cigarettes and pastry consumed. Recovering alcoholics often replace the alcohol with other substances to raise their blood sugar level. Some former drug addicts say that they use candy to help relieve their desire for drugs.

Over the years we have received many letters from recovering alcoholics and other substance abusers. It is fascinating to hear about their discovery that so many of their problems that had been attributed to their personality were actually caused by their faulty body chemistry, not their personality. The anger, internal unrest, clouds over their brain, mood swings, and anxiety disappeared after getting their blood sugar stable.

Is it any wonder it's a common occurrence for us to receive letters and orders for copies of the Low Blood Sugar Handbook to be sent to other recovering substance abusers.

All LBS people, be they substance abusers or not, suffer anxiety which is possibly caused by the release of excessive adrenalin and its effects on the cells. Excessive adrenalin is released when the blood sugar drops (due to drinking alcohol or eating the incorrect foods or not eating) as a result of the brain sending out a chemical message to the adrenal glands to release adrenalin. The adrenalin stimulates the liver to release glucose which is sent to the cells. This whole process may take only moments to occur. For certain the human body is magnificent and beautiful in how it can achieve these many vital functions. However, there is one nasty side effect, the excess adrenalin causes intolerable anxiety.

Psychological Problems

The symptoms displayed by a low blood sugar sufferer are often the same as those associated with emotional disturbance and the person is given medication or institutionalized. In various studies it has been found that many psychiatric patients, particularly those diagnosed schizophrenic, are really hypoglycemics. After being properly diagnosed (See chapter 3), these individuals improved immensely when given the proper diet and support. Many were eventually discharged on no, or very little medication. Low blood sugar is not a panacea, some would say if you're nuts, you're nuts. But until you can get your blood sugar straightened out, it's hard to tell if the nuttiness is due to LBS or to real psychiatric problems. A good question to ponder is, are there crazy people or just people acting crazy and for what reason?

If you have read this far and have started to get the impression that we are trying to sell you a cure-all for all of America's ills, you are right—to a degree. But we don't mean this as a medical witch hunt or a nutritional crusade. All we are trying to do is bring to light some of the things we have learned from our research and living with LBS. Let's assume that everything we have told you is 100% correct. Now just contemplate the amount of cultural breakdown and havoc, not to mention the medical bills and personal tragedies, that we have all experienced due to this still mysterious condition called low blood sugar.

Chapter 3

HOW TO DETERMINE IF YOU HAVE LOW BLOOD SUGAR

There is no sure fire, scientific method to determine whether a person has low blood sugar. But using the following methods (Tools) will give you a pretty definite conclusion.

TOOLS FOR DETERMINING LOW BLOOD SUGAR

There are three tools to use to determine if you have LBS:

1. Review of symptoms
2. 15-day food test
3. Glucose Tolerance Test—at best a poor tool

We believe that after doing 1 and 2 you'll find that 3 is not necessary.

Review of Symptoms for Evaluation

Comparing how you feel with the words on the symptom list is a very subjective experience. At best you with the suffering and the feelings can be the most suitable interpreter. Only you know the specifics of how you feel, and even you may not be able to put some of these feelings into words.

If you have several or more symptoms always or frequently, and/or many symptoms occasionally, we strongly recommend that you immediately get a thorough medical work up. Many of these symptoms can be indicative of conditions other than LBS.

If no other condition is found by the doctor, then LBS is possibly causing the symptoms. If another condition is diagnosed and treated and the symptoms persist, then again LBS should be considered.

We have set up the symptom list so you can do an inventory of your symptoms and their frequency before the 15-day food test and a review afterward.

The left columns are for your initial inventory. The columns to the right of the symptom list are for review. Check the appropriate letters:

A = Always
F = Frequently—once or more a week
O = Occasionally—once or more a month
N = Never

NOW

SYMPTOMS FOR EVALUATION

15 DAYS

A F O N

A F O N

Tiredness
Headaches
Drowsiness
Concentration problems
Irritability
Sleeping difficulties
Dizziness
Anxiety
Forgetfulness
Visual disturbances
Depression
Fainting/Blackouts
Cold hands and/or feet
Nervousness
Exhaustion
Shortness of breath
Temper outbursts
Sensitivity to light
Sensitivity to noise
Allergies
Muscle pains
Phobias (fears)
Crying spells
Antisocial behavior
Asocial behavior
Unsocial behavior
Suicidal thoughts and tendencies
Staggering
Craving for sweets
Unnecessary and excessive worrying
Mood swings (Dr. Jekyll & Mr. Hyde)
Nightmares
Digestive problems
Aching eye sockets
Lack of sex drive
Impotence
Indecisiveness
Heart palpitations

NOW					SYMPTOMS FOR EVALUATION	15 DAYS			
A	F	O	N			A	F	O	N
					Internal trembling				
					Mental confusion				
					Undue sweating				
					Bad breath				
					Negative thoughts and attitudes				
					Feeling of going mad, insane				
					Obestiy				
					Restlessness				
					Back ache and muscle pain				
					Sneezing				
					Waking up tired and exhausted				
					Arms and legs or body hurt when first rising in a.m.				
					Feel best after 7 p.m.				
					Gasping for breath				
					Sighing and yawning				
					Convulsions with no known cause				
					Premenstrual tension				
					"Motor Mouth" (constant talking)				
					Hand tremors				
					Accident prone				

Fifty eight symptoms are listed above. Count the responses to each letter and record the number for each below. This will afford you an easy visual aid to see your progress.

NOW	15 DAYS
A	A
F	F
O	O
N	N

Now you have a written record to help you determine the degree of your symptoms. You may want to make a copy of the list of your symptoms and their frequency to show your physician.

We have found at times that it is difficult to get a nonregulated low blood sugar person to relate to his symptoms. Sometimes he doesn't relate to them until he has been on our program for a while and the symptoms have begun to erode. This may be because he has had symptoms for so long that he assumes they are normal feelings, the way everyone feels all the time. Sometimes, too, after a symptom leaves a person he doesn't remember having it until he is reminded. A classic example is a person who has been getting headaches regularly for years, then goes on our program and eventually realizes the headaches are gone when asked if he still gets them.

15-Day Food Test

Other than following the Krimmel Program in Chapter 4, the 15-day food test is the most effective means for determining if you have functional LBS.

The underlying principle of the 15-day food test is to eat as few unrefined carbohydrates as possible, and to eat no refined carbohydrates, and see if you feel any better at the end of the test period. This is *not* a "cure all" period. By no means expect a 100% improvement. But by the end of 15-days you should notice some definite percentage of change. This improvement is an indication that your previous eating habits were detrimental to you and suggests that you may have LBS.

If after the 15-days you notice some definite positive differences you should plan to follow the Krimmel Program (Chp. 4), begin with the third week. It is also a good idea to mention your improvement to your doctor.

Please take special note that it is quite possible you may have negative reactions such as headaches, or excessive nervousness or upset stomach, or sleeping difficulty, etc. during the 15-days. We have found people have "withdrawal symptoms" from going off various carbohydrates and stimulants—just as people suffer when they first go off cigarettes. But the lifetime benefits are worth the initial discomfort.

However, it is the overall percentage of improvement you make during the period that is significant, not the intrusion of the withdrawal symptoms. You must keep these separate in your interpretation of the events. The withdrawal symptoms serve a significant benefit, they clearly point out that your body chemistry is reacting to not receiving the foodstuffs and stimulants that were harmful to you.

The 15-day food test consists of eating mostly protein foods, a few complex carbohydrate foods and no coffee, tea, alcohol, sodas or sugar in any form. (If you find you can't abstain from alcohol—you have a problem, call AA.) Also, it is of utmost importance that your 3 primary meals are moderate in amount and supplemented by snacks between meals. This helps to give your body a constant, even supply of blood sugar throughout the day.

Following are the only foods allowed during the 15-days:

Fowl, fish, meats—all types but with no breading or sauces. No lunch meats, hot dogs, sausages, scrapple or meats with fillers.
Eggs—any style.
Cheese—cheddar and swiss.
Vegetables—asparagus, green and wax beans, green peppers, raw mung bean sprouts, beet greens, broccoli, cauliflower, mushroom, tomatoes, celery, cucumbers, lettuce, onions, radishes, spinach, watercress.

Fruits—none.

Desserts—none.

Fats and oils—butter, soft margarine, vegetable oil spreads, and vegetable oil.

Bread, bread products, crackers, cereals—none.

Condiments—salt, pepper, vinegar and any spice that has no sugar added.

Beverages—water, seltzer water, clear broth.

Plain yogurt—may flavor with cinnamon or other desirable spice.

Sample Menu and Schedule—use only as a guide, eat as many different foods as you desire from the above list. Eat as large a quantity of vegetables as you wish.

6am Snack—¾ cup yogurt while sitting on edge of bed, then lie back and meditate for 3–4 minutes; for circulatory exercise, flex fingers, toes, arms and legs ten times each. Then get up and eat breakfast immediately. Don't get dressed.

6:15 Breakfast—eggs any style and/or serving of meat
vegetables if desired
8 oz. glass water

6:30 Shower, dress and get on with your day

8:00 Snack—1 stalk celery with one 1" sq. cheddar cheese

9:45 Snack—½ cup mung bean sprouts with ¼ cup plain yogurt

11:30 Lunch—tuna chunks, tomato slices, lettuce with vinegar and oil
raw or cooked cauliflower
8 oz. glass water

2:00 Snack—raw or cooked broccoli

4:15 Snack—2 oz. cooked chicken

6:30 Dinner—consomme
broiled flounder
green beans with mushrooms
asparagus
8 oz. glass of water

11:00 Snack just before getting into bed—¾ cup plain yogurt

During these 15-days eat a snack every 1½ hours between breakfast and lunch and every 2 hours between lunch and dinner. You are to avoid bread, flour products, sugar or anything containing it, fruits and juices. Eat only the foods listed above. Stay away from dietetic foods because they usually have some form of sugar, even when they claim to be "sugar free." Also, if you smoke, try to cut down and stopping would even be better.

The conscientious pursuit of this 15-day food test is imperative. You have a clean shot at being able to make a noticeable improvement in a very short period of time. You must make a fair bargain and try not to feel sorry for yourself about what you are "giving up." Instead, focus your mind's eye on our mutual objective—getting a specific measure of improvement on how you feel and function. Chances are that if you have read this far and have maintained an interest you have been putting up with quite a bit of pain and discomfort in your life. Take this opportunity to get a handle on some comfort and eventually some pleasure for yourself.

A frame of mind you may want to adopt is—imagine yourself in a life boat in the middle of the Atlantic waiting to be rescued. You have only the food and beverages we have permitted on the 15-day food program. How threatened would you feel about starving or how choosy would you be about having only these items to eat? Need I say more!?

For once in your life, be the one who is going to be able to take control of the pain and discomfort you have been living with for so long. *Do it with a spirit of 100%*—you won't believe the results—try it—you'll love it!

The Glucose Tolerance Test

What Is a Glucose Tolerance Test?

The Glucose Tolerance Test (GTT) measures the amount of sugar (glucose) in your blood at specific intervals. It shows how the body utilizes sugar. It is usually used to determine diabetes and hypoglycemia.

Reasons For Not Having a Glucose Tolerance Test

The GTT is time consuming and stressful and many times does not say unequivocally that you have LBS when actually you do. Why go through all that when the best means of testing is by following the 15 Day Food Test and see if your symptoms decrease or lessen in severity. If you feel improved, then follow the Krimmel Program.

Many people with so called "normal" GTT results experience severe symptoms while there are those with LBS test results who experience no symptoms. Imagine you've been through all kinds of tests and told there is nothing wrong with you even though you continue to have a variety of symptoms. You decide to take the GTT before changing your eating habits and according to your physician the test result are "normal." What may be considered normal results may not be normal for you. Your body may not be able to function properly with a blood sugar level that is not considered low enough to be diagnosed as low blood sugar. You may be one of those individuals who does not fit into the scientific standards that have been adopted for LBS but you suffer anyway. So what's left for you to do but try the LBS program and see if it helps relieve your symptoms? So why take the GTT?

Look at it another way, assume that you had a collection of symptoms that are on the symptom list, you followed the 15 days food test and the symptoms were significantly relieved. Would your next step be to get a GTT? Our answer is No! Our reasoning is, suppose you take the GTT and the results indicate you have LBS. What are you going to do other than continue following a LBS program to stabilize your blood sugar and live happily ever after. On the other hand, suppose the GTT results indicate you don't have LBS. Aren't you going to continue following a LBS program anyway since the 15 day test relieved your symptoms. So why take a GTT?

You must remember one vital point, if you suffer from a collection of symptoms, your only interest is in getting rid of those symptoms. And the only way to do that if you have functional LBS is to follow a LBS program, not take a GTT!

However, if you decide, for whatever reason, to take the GTT, please read the following sections on the GTT very carefully.

How Is a Glucose Tolerance Test Given?

It is vital that this test is given over a 6 hour period rather than a 3, 4, or 5 hour period. Many individuals' sugar does not drop until the 4th to 6th hour and this would be missed in a shorter test. If a doctor refuses to give a 6 hour test, find a doctor who will. This test should only be given after the doctor has taken a complete medical history, given a complete medical examination and heard a description of your symptoms. Be absolutely sure to inform the doctor of any and all medications you take, including aspirin and mention if you are pregnant.

The test is usually started in the morning after you have fasted (nothing to eat) for 10 to 12 hours. A sample of blood (fasting blood sugar) is drawn from your arm and then you are given a glucose (sugar) solution to drink. In a half hour blood will again be drawn and a urine sample requested. (In diabetes sugar may show up in the urine.) After that blood and urine samples will be taken on the hour for the next 5½ hours.

During the test no tobacco, chewing gum, food or drink, except water, is allowed.

If you have any symptoms or adverse effects during the test, write them down along with the time they occurred. When you have the test results you and your doctor should compare your reactions during the test to your blood sugar levels at the time of the reactions.

How to Interpret the Results of the Glucose Tolerance Test

To have a better understanding of the results of the GTT, here's some background. A normal fasting blood sugar is usually between 80 to 120 mg. Following a meal the blood sugar may rise to around 140 mg. If it goes to 170 or higher it is considered abnormal and the person should be checked for diabetes (hyperglycemia). For LBS (hypoglycemia) there is no specific number which can be used for a conclusive diagnosis.

In order for a doctor to make a correct diagnosis of hypoglycemia, he must be able to read the test results accurately. This is not easy to do unless the doctor has been specifically trained in this area because of the many differences in the sugar curves of hypoglycemia. Many doctors who do not specifically relate to this area feel that to be a hypoglycemic your blood sugar must fall lower than 65 mg. However, that isn't actually the case. Each person must be treated as an individual, what is low for one person is not necessarily low for another. It has been shown that some people have severe reactions even though their blood sugar never went below 75 mg.

There are two important dimensions to interpreting the GTT for LBS. These may be looked at separately or together.

1. It is not how low your blood sugar goes but *how fast you go to the low.* Your sugar may drop rapidly from 180 to 90 mg. over a one hour period and possibly cause more problems than slowly dropping from 110 to 50 mg. over a 2 to 3 hour period. Even though the 90 mg. reading is within the "normal range" the effects may be severe because the sugar dropped so rapidly where as the 50 mg. reading is in the "abnormal" range but because the drop was so slow the reaction may not be as severe, if any.
2. Again it is not how low your sugar goes but *how long it remains below your fasting level.* It may drop to 45 mg. but if it returns to your fasting level in an hour you may not notice it or have only mild symptoms. Whereas if the sugar dropped to 65 mg. and remains there for a few hours your symptoms may be much more severe, even though you didn't drop as low but because you took so long before returning to your fasting level. From this we can see that there are no set numbers to be used to diagnose hypoglycemia.

Be absolutely certain to get a copy of the results of your GTT. Make a graph of the results relating to the blood sugar values at the related times. The blank graph below can be used.

Your body needs a proper supply of blood sugar at all times for your brain and body to function adequately and efficiently. If you keep track of how you feel during the test, you can compare your feelings with your blood sugar levels represented on the graph. Also see how your graph compares to the two important dimensions listed above and to the graphs on the following pages.

Helpful Hints for Taking the GTT

Following are some helpful hints for making the test as pleasant as possible. Have some reading material or hand work to occupy your

Sample Graphs

The following graphs represent an overview of various common glucose tolerance test results.

NORMAL
Glucose Tolerance Curves
These are considered normal curves because of the following factors:

- Fasting levels are between 80 mg. and 120 mg.
- Curves do not go above 170 mg.
- Return to or near their fasting levels and remain there.
- No severe drops within a short period of time.

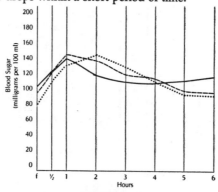

DIABETES
Glucose Tolerance Curves
These are considered diabetic curves because of the following factors:

- Curves go above 170 mg.
- Curves never drop to their fasting levels.

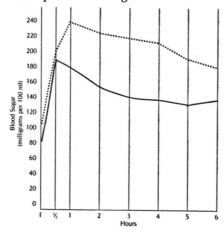

HYPOGLYCEMIA (LBS)
Glucose Tolerance Curves

These are considered hypoglycemic curves because of one or more of the following factors:

- Curves fall below their fasting levels.
- Curves stay below the fasting level for an extended period of time.
- Curves have severe percentage of drop in a short period of time.

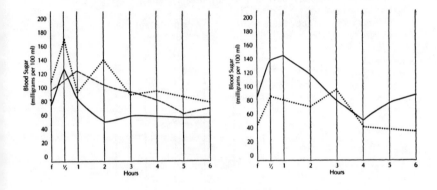

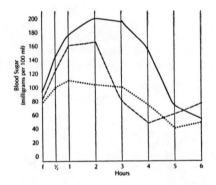

MODIFIED HYPOGLYCEMIA (LBS)
Flat Glucose Tolerance Curves
This is considered modified hypoglycemia because:

- Curves do not rise or fall appreciably.
- Curves do not rise to a normal level.
  Typically a person with this curve feels trapped and complains of boredom, loss of zest and fatigue. His lifestyle tends to be one of no substance and he has a feeling of no escape or refuge.

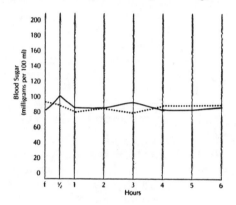

BLANK GRAPH
Use this to chart your glucose tolerance test results.   11/18/81

B_SD

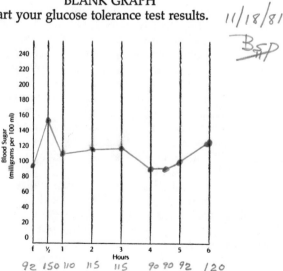

92 150 110   115   115   90 90 92   120

time. Take walks around the area if possible to relax you and to help make the situation more normal. Lie down only if you feel the need to. If the drawing of blood by one technician is too uncomfortable, ask for another technician to draw it. Pain and/or fear may increase your adrenal activity, which may interfere with your test results. (If possible, check with friends and nurses to discover a skillful and gentle technician.)

Since you will not be eating for many hours and your sugar level may go low this can be a very stressful test. Make plans for someone to drive you home afterwards if the test is done as an outpatient. If you are going by public transportation have someone with you. A friend or relative should be with you during the test. Have a snack (orange, apple, cheese etc.) with you to eat as soon as the test is over. Do not drive or do anything dangerous until after you have had a proper meal and rest.

Anyone with a history of passing out or seizures may want to have the test done at a hospital laboratory rather than a private laboratory.

UNDERSTANDING THE PHYSICIAN'S ROLE— DOCTOR, PATIENT RELATIONSHIP

Generally speaking we would like very much to simply tell you that it isn't necessary to go to a physician but to just read books about hypoglycemia and follow their instructions. However, that would be pure folly because your symptoms may be related to a condition other than hypoglycemia or your hypoglycemia may be caused by an organic problem that needs attention. These organic problems could be related to your pancreas, liver, pituitary gland, adrenal glands, etc. So, in the final analysis you must consult a physician.

If there is one thing that becomes certain to a hypoglycemic it is the fact that he must master the art of dealing with physicians. If you have any quantity of symptoms from the symptom list, you most likely have been put through the frustration more than once that the medical camp too often offers to the hypoglycemic. A harsh reality which all hypoglycemics must face is that they must become their own best friend and pseudo physician in dealing with their condition as a low blood sugar sufferer.

However, as we stated before you must utilize various medical resources. That being the case we have set down some guidelines you may find helpful when doing so. In addition most libraries have books on how to choose and deal with your doctor, we strongly recommend you reading them.

Types of Physicians

The types of physicians you would consider seeing for diagnosing conditions related to your symptoms are listed below in alphabetical order, not in order of importance or anything else.

Endocrinologist—deals with diseases of the endocrine glands i.e., pancreas, thyroid, pituitary, pineal, parathyroid, thymus and adrenals.

General practitioner (GP) or Family practitioner—has general knowledge of routine health maintenance. Will usually refer you to a specialist if he does not feel knowledgeable enough about your condition.

Internist—treats nonsurgical problems located between the head and the pelvis.

Of the three types of physicians listed, the endocrinologist is the more favorable physician in our opinion. He is often considered by his peers to be an excellent diagnostician, which is really what you are looking for. Even if he may not give credibility to LBS there is a high possibility he may find a condition aggravating the LBS such as adrenal insufficiency, liver condition, etc. Of course the best of all worlds would be an endocrinologist who would give credibility to the existence of hypoglycemia whether you have it or not.

Making a Choice

Things to consider when choosing a physician:

- Be certain the physician is affiliated with a very good hospital because this is often a strong indicator the physician is well qualified in his area. But let us caution you, this is not 100% fool proof.
- Check with the doctor, hospital and local medical association for his schooling and experience.
- Talk with the doctor's patients and coworkers at the hospital (nurses and technicians) for their opinion of his capability. When doing this, be aware the personalities may influence their responses and be subjective rather than objective.
- The location of the doctor's office should not take an excessive amount of time to reach.
- Consider the age of the physician. If you are young and want the same doctor for your lifetime then you would rather have a young physician. On the other hand maybe an older physician won't live as long as you but his experience may outweigh his age factor. Yet another factor is that a young physician may have more up-to-date information and knowledge. All of these thoughts you must weigh and come up with your own personal decision. Good luck!
- Call the physician and speak to him about his feelings on hypoglycemia, does he or doesn't he believe it to be a legitimate, plausible and acceptable health condition, independent of diabetes. Here are some other questions to ask the doctor.
    - How long a GTT do you order? If the answer is anything less than 6 hours, it is inadequate.
    - What diet do you recommend for LBS? If the answer is to only stay off sweets or drink a coke when feeling down, that is a very poor answer.

How low does one's blood sugar have to go to have LBS? If the answer is a specific number rather than individual results, it is a poor and inadequate answer.

Does he do a complete body chemistry work-up? The answer should be yes.

Will he treat you for your symptoms without a GTT?

These questions are to be done as the last item in choosing your physician, only after you are contented with all other feedback you have gotten. Our concern is that you don't fall into the hands of a physician who specializes in preying on hypoglycemics, unfortunately there are some around. Your only protection against them is adequate knowledge—and the only way to get adequate knowledge is to read, read, read, think, reason and stay alert!

Physician's Role and Responsibilities

It is the physician's responsibility to be interested in his patients' well-being and give them the best care that he is capable of giving. In order to do this he must be willing to practice the art of healing. The art of healing requires the following attributes.

He must be:

- An effective listener—listen for the concepts (ideas) that are trying to be stated, not just the words that are being uttered. Non-medical people often have a limited resource of words to use in explaining how they feel. Too often doctors expect laymen to be able to use medical terminology.
- Open minded to and understand all health-care schools of thought—such as the importance nutrition can play in maintaining good health.
- Able to ask effective questions—the questions should relate to all aspects of your life, physical, mental and spiritual and then he should relate the answers to each other. For instance, a certain mental or physical feeling may be a side effect of a medication you're taking or some symptoms may be related to recent family stress, a death or illness in the family.
- A creative thinker—you should be seen as an individual, not as a stereotype, you should be viewed as a creature comprised of a body, mind and spirit, not just a one dimensional creature having only a body. In his thinking about your symptoms his vision should be wide spectrum rather than tunnel vision.
- An effective test selector—not do unnecessary tests.
- Capable of interpreting test results and relating them to other results and/or symptoms.
- Up to date on nutritional information and use it.
- Able to diagnose accurately.
- Able to treat and prescribe properly.
- Willing to use consultants such as other physicians and dieticians.

How to Prepare to Go to the Physician

In order for your visit to the physician to be most productive it is necessary for you to be prepared to ask questions and to answer the questions you will be asked. Following are some hints to help you prepare.

Make a memo list including:
- symptoms that occur frequently and occasionally
- how you feel at different times of day
- names of medications you take, including vitamins
- conditions being treated by other physicians
- past medical history with dates such as operations and major illnesses

You may want to take your spouse or friend along for support and to verify your situation.

Call physician's office to check if he is there and if his appointments are on schedule—this can save you time, stress, aggravation and money.

How to Talk and Act with a Physician

The number one role of a physician is to be a keen and discerning listener. You must be certain that he listens to what you are saying and not be distracted by and/or misled by your healthy physical appearance (if you have a healthy appearance). You must make him aware that the way you may look physically is not always indicative of the way you feel. Too often, because of cultural tradition we go to our physician's office dressed in our "Sunday best." Sometimes we even smile and practice our very best of social gestures when in actuality we feel as if we can barely walk. Maybe the best way to go is acting the way you usually feel, don't put up a special front or on a smiling false face. Show your real self, otherwise you will be sending two messages to the physician. One verbal and one physical and they may not jibe.

While you are describing your symptoms give the doctor a list of your symptoms which occur always and frequently and use your copy to aid yourself in describing your problems. We repeat, remember your symptoms list is just words on paper, they must be dramatized and explained sufficiently for the doctor to get an understanding of how these symptoms fit you and affect you as a specific individual.

Let us tell you of a possible entrapment that is very likely to occur when you go to a physician. Usually there is some degree of fear or apprehension attached to going to a physician. When this occurs the adrenal glands are activated and stimulate the liver to release glucose which often gives you a mental and physical "pick up" and when you are with the physician you may feel considerably better than usual. Until we learned this concept we couldn't understand why Ed acted like he was at the Academy Awards rather than in a doctor's office. Here he was, telling the doctor about all these symptoms he suffered on a regular basis and looking as if he had just won an oscar. What with flashing his pearlies, shaking hands with the doctor and looking like a million, is it any wonder the doctor didn't give credibility to his symptoms?

If at any time during your visit with the physician you see him getting a haze over his eyes, becoming disinterested, impatient or looking at his watch as if he is in a hurry, you better decide if you are with a person who is willing to listen and take a sincere and healthful interest in you. If you feel the slightest tinge of the answer being no, our experience is that you better get your hat and leave because you are in a nonhelping situation. We have yet to meet a hypoglycemic who hasn't been in this situation at least a couple of times. Don't let it distract you or get you upset. It's just the reality of how the medical camp, to a very large percentage, looks upon hypoglycemia. It hasn't anything to do with you as an individual. How can a doctor be expected to understand something which he hasn't been taught or is not interested in?

When the time comes, whether your diagnosis be low blood sugar or another condition, ask your doctor to explain your diagnosis, medications, treatment and tests to you in layman's terms so you can completely understand what your condition is, what causes it, how it will be treated and for how long, is there any pain involved in the condition, treatment or test and are there any side effects that may occur due to the medication or treatment. Also what will the cost be.

Ask if the treatment will cure the condition or just control it. Also are there any choices of treatment and why has he chosen the particular one. Can he suggest any books to read on the condition and its treatment. If the condition is severe or prolonged, are there any support groups you can contact?

Some Important Medical Tests

There are three immediate rewards for learning more about medical testing:

1. You will be able to communicate more thoroughly with your physician.
2. Your physician will be compelled to function more competently and creatively.
3. You will be more discriminating about the competence of your physician and his willingness to be helpful and work with you.

For more information on medical tests, contact your lending library system for books pertaining to medical tests and procedures, there are many available. If not available at your library, ask them to order the books for you.

The various tests that we have listed are but a few of the most important tests to be considered when having a complete medical work-up. Our main purpose for listing these is to give you an introduction to the idea of thinking about tests and their meanings. We strongly urge you to make every possible effort to familiarize yourself with as many medical tests as possible.

Complete blood count (CBC)—measures the number of red blood cells (4½ to 5 million per cubic millimeter), hemoglobin (necessary for carrying oxygen), and white blood cells (5 to 9 thousand per cmm.). White blood cells increase during infection.

Erythrocyte sedimentation rate (ESR)—how far the red cells sink in a test tube in 1 hour. In a disease condition the red cells sink more rapidly than when healthy, this is not related to a specific disease.

Blood chemistry—tests with one blood sample include information on:

- Cholesterol and triglycerides—deals with fat metabolism
- Albumin total protein—concerns liver function
- Globulins—measured with albumin, related to body defense mechanism
- Uric acid—deals with kidney function
- Bilirubin—relates to liver function
- LDH—relates to liver function
- Alkaline phosphate—relates to liver function
- SGOT—increased amount indicative of heart disease. If increased along with SGPT, indicative of liver disease.
- SGPT—increased amount indicative of liver disease
- BUN—blood urea nitrogen, increased level may indicate kidney disease
- Creatinine—indicates kidney functioning
- Calcium & Phosphorous—measured together
- Chlorides—increase in nephritis, anemia and cardiac disease; decreased in fevers and diabetes
- Potassium—may be low if taking diuretics, having chronic diarrhea, kidney disease or overproduction of corticosteroids.

T-3, T-4, TSH—relates to thyroid functioning

Urine test

24 hour urine collection for 17 hydrox and 17 Keto steroids—analyzed for specific hormones related to the adrenal glands and gonads.

Diet analysis—review of eating habits in relation to quantity and quality.

Glucose tolerance test—determines how your body handles carbohydrates. Ideal for diagnosing diabetes but not hypoglycemia (LBS).

It is not possible to test for the amount of all the vitamins and minerals present in our bodies. Also all of the normal ranges have not been decided. There are however some blood and urine tests which can determine the level of certain vitamins and minerals in our bodies.

It must be remembered that deficiencies are sometimes caused by poor absorption rather than by not ingesting an adequate diet.

Blood tests can be done for the following vitamins and minerals:

- Vitamin A
- Vitamin D—done by measuring the alkaline phosphatase, calcium and phosphorus in blood.
- Vitamin K—done by measuring rate of blood clotting in test tube.
- Vitamin E   · Cooper
- Vitamin B_1 · Magnesium
- Folic Acid   · Manganese
- Vitamin B_{12} · Zinc
- Vitamin C   · Lead
- Chromium

Urine tests can be done for the following vitamins and minerals:

- Vitamin B_2
- Vitamin B_3—done with 6 hour urine sample
- Vitamin B_6—done with 24 hour urine sample
- Sodium
- Cadmium
- Arsenic—done with 24 hour urine sample
- Mercury—done with 24 hour urine sample

SUFFERERS BEWARE!!!

Be sure to use the whole wheel, not just half

It is imperative that the information in this book, *especialy chapters 5, 6, 8 and 9,* be kept ever present for immediate recall and use. We, the authors, literally spent thousands of hours learning, conceptualizing and drafting the tools of this handbook. All the information we worked so hard to deliver is not helping you if you only read the book once and then put it aside, thinking you'll remember what to do or lend it to someone else.

Remember, this is a handbook. It is to be used daily, read *again and again and again to help you retain the concepts so you can use them to regulate your blood sugar.* Even we have to keep reading material about LBS in order to stay sharp—*and we wrote the handbook!*

If you want a friend or relaitve to have a copy of the handbook, *we will mail them a copy . . . autographed.* See order form in back of book.

Chapter 4

THE KRIMMEL PROGRAM WHAT TO DO IF YOU HAVE LOW BLOOD SUGAR

This is the most important part of this book. It doesn't matter what you call your condition or who knows you have it, or how you found out you have low blood sugar or how long or how much you suffered before finding out you have it. It all goes for nought if you don't know what to do about it!

Too often we have heard from LBS victims that they had been diagnosed many years earlier but were never told the specifics of what and how to maintain a stable blood sugar level. Too often the doctor passes over the condition and its suffering as if a human being were not living inside the skin of the body in front of him. Or the LBS sufferer is told such misdirected solutions that in some respects it would have been better had the doctor not diagnosed LBS at all.

So, no matter what your past experience or how you feel about what you've been told—don't let it stand in your way now. Put it all behind you and rest assured that here is a program that will mend you.

Don't waste a moment—start now—today is the beginning of the rest of your life—live it without the suffering of LBS.

The Krimmel Program has four specific and vital dimensions:

1. Food ethic
2. Exercise
3. Sleep, rest and relaxation
4. Fun and laughter

Think of a square—each of its sides are equally important in maintaining its strength. Likewise with the Krimmel Program—each of its four dimensions is equally important in reaching and maintaining a stable blood sugar and body chemistry.

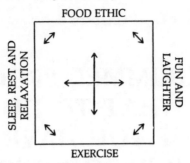

As the arrows indicate, each of these four vital dimensions is interwoven. You must consider each equally important and learn to see how they are dependent on one another. There is one other dimension which is required for your personal well-being and it would be in the center of the square and subsequently be the center of your life. That, of course, is your personal spiritual enrichment.

You must also see these four dimensions as a staircase to a stable blood sugar and body chemistry.

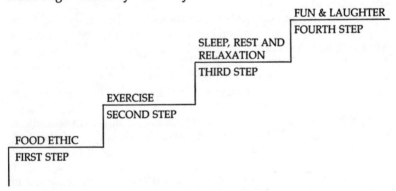

NOW GET STEPPING! ! ! ! !

Our opinion is that you have very little chance of having fun and laughter (enjoying life) if you are eating the wrong foods. Sure, you may have lots of excitement—from the delights of strawberry shortcake to the excitement you may get from alcohol. But to have the true delights of living and a quality type of fun and laughter you must first stabilize your body chemistry. That being the case you must start somewhere—and our suggestion has always been to start with the food ethic.

Shortly after you begin your exercise program, sleep, rest and relaxation will easily be accomplished along with the fun and laughter.

We are certain you couldn't possibly have fun and laughter if you're still getting kicked in the brain by lows in your blood sugar day in and day out. You probably won't be able to get stability with your sleep, rest and relaxation either. So—see clearly the approach we are recommending and give it a step by step try.

A question most often asked is, "How soon will I begin feeling better once I start the Krimmel Program 100%?" We have found that some symptoms may clear up as early as 10 to 15 days. While others may take longer. But the majority of your symptoms should be gone by the end of the third month—providing you followed the Krimmel Program 100%. Get stepping!!

FOOD ETHIC

Although the word cell has only four letters and goes largely unnoticed most of the time, cells are the building blocks of your body and all other living substances. Everything in your body is made from various types of cells; blood cells, bone cells, muscle cells, nerve cells, skin cells, etc. The cells in your body are what you are all about in every aspect. All functional activities of the body are carried on by cells. Your body functions only as well as your cells are functioning and your cells function well only if they are receiving all the nutrients (water, vitamins, minerals, protein, carbohydrates, fat) they need to keep them healthy. It's that simple!

When following the Krimmel Program, guess what you are trying to change and stabilize? You guessed it, the cells in your body! If you can change how your cells are functioning to the degree that is required to rid yourself of the symptoms you have been experiencing, you will begin feeling stable. It's that simple! You should endeavor to stabilize your body chemistry by keeping your cells from over-reacting. In other words, keep too much insulin and adrenalin from being released.

Every time you eat something it will have a direct and significant influence on how your cells function. Eating should not be simply a matter of satisfying your taste buds, but rather a process of taking in the best nutrients for the cells in your body to use to stay healthy and full of energy. You eat plant and/or animal cells to supply nutrients to the cells in your body. Many foods (white flour and/or sugar products, ice cream, sodas, etc.) that satisfy the taste buds have very few if any nutrients. This is one reason the Krimmel Program suggests avoiding certain types of foods.

In order to improve your LBS condition, as well as your general health, it is helpful to learn, understand and use some food chemistry concepts. Since food chemistry is directly related to body chemistry, the more you know about both, the better prepared you will be to take care of yourself. Naturally the more you learn, the more interesting and beneficial this type of information can become in managing your own well-being.

If you did not understand the last four paragraphs, right down to the cells of the marrow of your bones, then you are never going to get the total benefit of the concepts in this book. Subsequently, reread, and think about the four paragraphs and discuss them with others. For the past 15 years we've been thinking and working on these concepts and you probably won't find them written anywhere else. Just bear with the culture and hopefully it will soon catch up, in the meantime you have to understand them on your own.

For a dramatic demonstration of how cells react to various conditions, take three flourishing plants and set them in the same ideal location; 1 plant don't water, 1 plant water as needed, 1 plant water and fertilize as needed. Watch what happens to the plants over an extended period of time. If the plant's cells don't receive what they need, the cells degenerate and therefore the plant degenerates. If the cells receive everything they need the cells flourish and therefore the plant flourishes. The cells in your body react the same way, so be certain to care for your cells by giving them everything they need. That's what the Krimmel Program is all about.

Foods are comprised of carbohydrates, proteins and fats. Most foods have a combination of all three, for example:

Food Item	Carbohydrate	Protein	Fat
4 ozs. plain low fat yogurt	8 grams	6 grams	2 grams
⅓ cup oatmeal	18 grams	5 grams	2 grams
1 baked potato with skin	51 grams	5 grams	trace
½ grapefruit	10 grams	1 grams	trace
3 ozs. roasted chicken breast	0 grams	27 grams	3 grams
¼ cup almonds	7 grams	7 grams	17 grams
1 cup cooked broccoli	4.6 grams	2.6 grams	trace
½ Avocado	6 grams	2 grams	15 grams

Carbohydrates—starches and sugars. They are the chief source of energy for all body functions and are necessary to assist in the digestion and assimilation of other foods. There are complex and simple carbohydrates. Complex carbohydrates are those foods comprised of mainly starch such as vegetables, nuts, seeds and grains while simple carbohydrates are those high in sugar such as fruits. All starches and sugars are converted to glucose during digestion and absorbed into the blood stream as glucose (blood sugar). The lower the percentage of carbohydrate content, the more favorable it is for hypoglycemics. The lower the percentage, the less sugar there will be made by the body.

The percentage of carbohydrate content is found by adding the weights of protein, fat, carbohydrate and water for the specific food and dividing the total of these into the weight of the carbohydrates.

For example, a raw, unpeeled cucumber has .9 grams of protein, .1 grams of fat, 3.4 grams of carbohydrate and 95.1 grams of water. That totals 99.5 grams which is divided into 3.4 grams of carbohydrates and equals 3% carbohydrate content.

Under the section, Foods To Eat For the Rest of Your Life, vegetables and fruits are listed according to percentage of carbohydrate content.

Proteins—found in all living things; in such foods as cheese, meat, fowl, fish, shellfish, dairy products, eggs, grains and nuts. One of the most important elements for the maintenance of good health and vitality and is of primary importance in the growth and development of all body cells.

Fats—butter, margarine and vegetable oils make up the classic group of fat we consume. They are needed for energy and the utilization of fat soluble vitamins A, D, E and K. Also needed for steroid production. Fats slow the stomach's secretion of hydrochloric acid which increases the time needed for digestion, thereby giving a longer period of satisfaction after a meal.

Eat Low Protein, High Complex Carbohydrate and Low Fat

The usual diet recommended for low blood sugar (LBS) is high protein, low carbohydrate and moderate fat, called the Seale Harris diet. It is named for the doctor who first discovered LBS in 1923 and advised this diet for treating the condition. However, in recent years many studies indicate that eating a low protein, high complex carbohydrate diet of vegetables, grains, seeds, nuts and fruits is much better. Subsequently let's be done with the idea that a LBS sufferer should eat a high protein, low carbohydrate, and moderate fat diet. Medical science has shown that too much protein and fat is detrimental to one's overall health. Therefore, you should be following a low protein, high complex carbohydrate, and low fat food ethic. Your total daily calorie intake should be comprised of:

50–65% from carbohydrates; those listed under Foods You May Eat
10–12% from proteins; those listed under Foods You May Eat
20–30% from fats, visible and invisible, mostly unsaturated fat

For example, for an 1800 calorie daily intake, the range of calories should be:

900 to 1170 calories from carbohydrates
180 to 216 calories from protein
360 to 540 calories from fat

None of your carbohydrates should come from those vegetables and fruits listed under vegetables and fruits to avoid later in this chapter.

Some people determine how much to eat by instinct while others wish to be academic and calculate how many calories from each category (protein, carbohydrate, fats) should be eaten. If you wish to calculate, just multiple the percentage times the total amount of daily calories to be eaten. For example, if you want to eat 1800 calories daily; for carbohydrate calories multiple .65 (65%) times 1800 calories = 1170 calories; for protein calories multiple .12 (12%) times 1800 = 216 calories; for fat calories multiple .20 (20%) times 1800 = 360 calories, for a total of 1746 calories.

Most grain products and frozen vegetables have the number of calories, grams of carbohydrates, protein and fat per serving listed on the container. To determine how many calories of each are in a serving, you need to multiple the grams of carbohydrate and protein times 4 because there are 4 calories in each gram of carbohydrate and protein. Each gram of fat has 9 calories so multiple 9 times the grams of fat listed. For example, a serving of oatmeal with ½ cup of 2% milk has:

24 grams of carbohydrate .... multiple 24 × 4 = 96 calories
9 grams of protein .... multiple 9 × 4 = 36 calories
4 grams of fat .... multiple 4 × 9 = 36 calories

The above are some of the keystone concepts in relation to understanding food chemistry and ultimately body chemistry. It may be worthwhile to spend some extra time learning about the carbohydrate, protein, and fat content of the foods you eat. Your body chemistry's health is directly related to the type, quality and quantity of food you eat.

In order to decide how much food or how many calories to eat daily, you must take into consideration your ideal weight, physical activity (work and exercise), age and gender. You should also be drinking 6 to 8 glasses of water a day.

See back of book for ordering information pertaining to food chemistry; carbohydrate, protein, fat and calorie content of foods.

LBS is aggravated by all forms of sugar (be it added or in fruit), starch, fast acting carbohydrates, stimulants (caffeine, nicotine) and additives such as monosodium glutamate (MSG), sulfites and, artificial flavoring, colorings and sweeteners.

Your food ethic (diet) will be comprised of slow acting (unrefined) carbohydrates, proteins and fats; no fast acting (refined) carbohydrates (sugars and white flour products) or stimulants. You will eat 3 moderate size meals a day supplemented by snacks at proper (timely) intervals between your main meals. You should eat something approximately every 1½ to 2 hours to maintain an even level of blood sugar.

A snack is to be "a snack," not a small meal, not too little and not too much. Sometimes it will also require your own good judgment to learn which type of snack is best for different times of the day.

This part of interpreting your body chemistry's needs can be learned only by you, you are the one receiving your body's messages (symptoms). We can give you some general ideas but you are the one who must do the fine tuning and become the fine musician in playing your body chemistry for its most stable worth. Keep practicing!

Remember, you're the only person in the world who can take charge of your well-being if you have LBS. Please take charge and learn—learn—learn, and read—read—read, get stable, it's great, but you must be the one who takes the interest and does it. Not your spouse, parent, friend, doctor, etc, etc. You are the only one who can take charge!

As we have noted, carbohydrates are vegetables, grains, seeds, nuts, and fruits. These foods in their natural states are slow acting carbohydrates. The farther away they get from their natural state the faster acting (refined) they become. For example, let us look at an apple. A whole uncooked apple is a slow acting carbohydrate—you must chew it thoroughly before it can be swallowed and then it has to be broken down further by stomach acids and intestinal juices before it can be absorbed through the intestinal wall. However if that apple were made into applesauce it would become a faster acting carbohydrate because the cooking has begun the chemical and mechanical breakdown and you don't have to chew it. There is less work for the stomach acids and intestinal juices, so it is absorbed faster. Apple juice is almost completely broken down and all you do is swallow it and it is absorbed very fast, therefore it is a fast acting carbohydrate. (An over simplified explanation)

Since carbohydrates are broken down into glucose, drinking apple juice or any fruit juice and some vegetable juices is almost like drinking sugar. The more refined or processed a food is the less work your digestive system has to do and the more quickly absorption takes place. It may be that some juices are starting to be absorbed into the blood stream in the mouth. The mouth has a rich supply of blood vessels and there is an enzyme called ptyalin in your saliva which begins to breakdown carbohydrates in your mouth. This ptyalin may be able to breakdown some of the juice molecules small enough so they can be absorbed through the mouth tissue into your blood stream rather than through the intestinal wall. Also, some more of the glucose molecules may be absorbed through the stomach wall. This would be putting glucose into the blood stream faster than if they all waited to be slowly absorbed through the intestinal wall.

Alcohol is another fast acting carbohydrate and it has to go through fewer chemical changes than sugar and therefore is the quickest source of energy. This may be why many LBS people become alcoholics, alcohol gives them that quick pick up they want and need.

But the pick up doesn't last long, so they have another drink and eventually they are chemically and physically hooked. Some people get hooked on candy or colas for their pick up—maybe partly because of taste.

A Secret Your Body Knows

We have mentioned before how the adrenals stimulate the liver to release glucose into the blood stream. The original use for this system was to help us when frightened or in danger. If we are in danger, the adrenal glands release adrenalin which stimulates the liver to release glucose and we get a quick supply of energy to defend ourselves from the danger. You have heard of people lifting a car off a loved one at a scene of an accident—well this is where their extra energy and strength comes from, of course that is an extreme example.

Another way the adrenals are stimulated is by the caffeine in coffee, tea, colas, chocolate and cocoa and the nicotine in tobacco products. Just think of the yo-yo effect this has on your body's systems. You drink a cup of coffee and/or have a cigarette, the adrenals are stimulated to release adrenalin, which stimulates the liver to release glucose, the pancreas releases insulin so the glucose can be utilized. When the glucose is first released you get a "pick up," but when it has been all utilized the blood sugar level falls and you feel the need for another "pick up"—so—more coffee or cigarettes and "up and down" your adrenals, liver and pancreas go until they may wear out or at least become exhausted and sluggish. They were not made for this kind of life, they were made to handle a slow, even supply of glucose that would be released from the digestion of slow acting carbohydrates.

The secret your body knows is whether it is getting the proper foods or not. And if it isn't it tells you so by sending you messages through the symptoms you get. A well balanced body chemistry keeps its secret well—you don't get any symptoms such as headaches, mood swings, sleeping problems, etc., etc., etc.

First Month of the Krimmel Program

Your main goal in the first month is to avoid all fast acting carbohydrates, sugars and stimulants completely. At the end of the month you will have gained many rewards for your 100% effort. You may be surprised to notice some positive changes in as few as 3 to 5 days. Many people rationalize that these positive feelings are due to something other than the way they are eating.

After the first month you will probably find yourself saying, *"I haven't felt this good since I was a child."* Some of the most common comments we have heard are:

- "I can think more clearly and my concentration span is longer."
- "I don't feel as if my brain is in a vise."
- "The cloud has been lifted from over my brain."
- "I have less trouble breathing."
- "I have more energy. I don't have that dragged-out feeling."
- "I have fewer mood swings and emotional outbursts."
- "Bright lights and loud noises don't annoy me now."

A word of caution—it is not always clear sailing. There will be times you'll wish you had never heard of the "Krimmel Program" and the next day you will thank your lucky stars for it. At times you will feel like you are dangling from a yo-yo and the next day you may feel like you are sitting on top of the world. Here are some additional phenomena that may occur off and on during the first 2 months of the program.

- Your symptoms are subject to becoming more severe at times.
- You may have headaches, sleeping problems or other symptoms you didn't have before.
- You may have periods when you have less energy than you did before you started.
- You may have periods of high energy. (Discipline yourself not to be overly active and don't make plans that depend on the high energy level, which may not last.)
- You may have periods of the blahs—don't feel good but don't feel bad.
- You may crave sugar, starches and/or stimulants.
- You may be hungry all the time.
- You may become demoralized due to various changes occurring and feel no progress is being made and want to abandon the program. This is the ideal time to review your progress with your copilot. (See Ch. 5)
- The phantom "I am cured" strikes—you start feeling very good and think you can eat and do what ever you want.

Some of the rewards for going through the above frustration are:

- You can handle situations you couldn't handle before—you won't lose control—or your temper—where you ordinarily did. You can perform a task you couldn't do before.
- You don't get headaches.
- No more severe mood swings.
- You know you are not crazy or a hypochondriac because now you know where your symptoms come from.
- Oh how sweet it is to be able to concentrate for a longer period of time.
- It's moved! Anxiety doesn't live here anymore!

Special Notes

It is most important that you limit yourself to no more than seven to eight hours sleep a night so your blood sugar doesn't dip too low from being without food for that time. It is proposed that the brain cells release substances early in the morning hours that make it very favorable and beneficial to start your day as close to 5:30 am as possible, 6:30–7 is somewhat okay but 8 is just too late. Of course if you work nights or evenings this is impossible, but you should still limit yourself to seven or eight hours of sleep.

Remember, moderation is usually the best policy in all of life, don't become a yogurt freak, protein freak, nut freak or a freak of any kind. Don't try to eat yourself out of the LBS condition by over eating or eating too frequently. Eating high quality foods at timely intervals is just as important as eating the correct foods; a small snack every 1½ hours between breakfast and lunch and a small snack every 2 hours between lunch and dinner with a snack at bedtime is ideal. Eating too much and/or too often may result in an excess of insulin being released which is one of the things you are trying to prevent.

Although the Krimmel Program is not a high protein food ethic, you will be eating a significant amount of protein for the first few weeks. After the first few weeks, you will gradually decrease the protein foods as you increase your carbohydrate foods. This is done to help your body adjust and make certain necessary changes.

The first month of the Krimmel Program is divided into weekly segments. Your food choices increase each week.

First Week

Eat only the foods listed.

Fowl—broiled or roasted turkey, chicken or duck. No gravy, filling or sauces.

Fish and shellfish—all, but no breading or sauces.

Meats—broiled, roasted or baked beef, veal, pork and lamb. No breading, gravies or sauces.

Eggs—any style.

Cereal—No more than 1 serving a day; Oat Bran or non instant Oatmeal, add a pat of butter or margarine and/or 1 Tbs. toasted wheat germ, sprinkled on top. Absolutely no form of sweetener is to be used.

Milk—to be used only for cereal and cooking.

Vegetables—alfalfa sprouts, asparagus, bamboo shoots, beet greens, broccoli, raw cabbage, cauliflower, celery, chives, collards, cucumber, dandelion greens, eggplant, endive, escarole, fennel, green beans, kale, kohlrabi, lettuce, mung bean sprouts, mushrooms, okra, olives, onions, parsley, sweet peppers, dill pickles, pimientos, radishes, swiss chard, tofu, soybean milk, spinach, tomatoes, turnips, turnip greens, watercress, yellow wax beans, zucchini.

Fruits—none.

Cheese—all cheeses, preferably low fat (no cheese spreads).

Yogurt—plain, low fat yogurt.

Bread, bread products, crackers, etc.—none.

Grains—wheat germ.

Fats and oils—butter, soft margarine, vegetable oil spreads, vegetable oils (canola preferable).

Beverages—water, seltzer water and clear broth.

Condiments—salt, pepper, lemon juice, mustard, horseradish, vinegar and all sugar free spices.

Tobacco products—tobacco usage should be reduced by 50% during the first week, for example—if you are using 20 cigarettes per day at the start of the Krimmel Program you should be smoking only 10 a day by the end of the first week. You will be very surprised how easy this is to accomplish after 2 or 3 days. It's due to the fact that you are stopping all other things that shoot up your body and brain. This is true with other tobacco products as well.

Sample Menu and Schedule—use only as a guide, eat as many different foods from the above list as you desire.

6am Snack, imperative, must be done every morning
¾ cup yogurt while sitting on edge of bed, then lie back and meditate for 3–4 minutes; for exercise, flex fingers, toes, arms and legs ten times each. Then get up and go to the bathroom.

6:15 Breakfast—scrambled egg(s) and or
1 cup cooked oat bran with small pat of butter or margarine & 1 Tbs. wheat germ sprinkled on top
½ cup milk on oat bran
8 oz. glass water

6:30 Shower, dress and get on with your day

8:00 Snack—1 stalk celery with one 1" sq. cheddar cheese

9:45 Snack—½ cup alfalfa sprouts with ¼ cup plain yogurt

11:30 Lunch—tuna chunks, tomato slices on lettuce with vinegar and oil olives
raw or cooked cauliflower
8 oz. glass water

2:00 Snack—raw or cooked broccoli

4:15 Snack—2 oz. cooked chicken

6:30 Dinner—consomme
broiled flounder
green beans with mushrooms
zucchini with tomatoes and onions
8 oz. glass of water

11:00 Snack, imperative, must be done every night just before getting into bed—¾ cup yogurt

Second Week

Eat only the foods listed.

Fowl—broiled or roasted turkey, chicken or duck. No gravy, filling or sauces.

Fish and shellfish—all but no breading or sauces.

Meats—broiled, roasted or baked beef, veal, pork and lamb. No breading, gravies or sauces.

Eggs—any style.

Cereal—No more than 1 serving a day; Oat Bran or non instant Oatmeal, add a pat of butter or margarine and/or 1 Tbs. toasted wheat germ, sprinkled on top. Absolutely no form of sweetener is to be used.

Milk—to be used only for cereal and cooking.

Vegetables—alfalfa sprouts, asparagus, bamboo shoots, beet greens, broccoli, raw cabbage, cauliflower, celery, chives, collards, cucumber, dandelion greens, eggplant, endive, escarole, fennel, green beans, kale, kohlrabi, lettuce, mung bean spouts, mushrooms, okra, olives, onions, parsley, sweet peppers, dill pickles, pimientos, radishes, swiss chard, tofu, soybean milk, spinach, tomatoes, turnips, turnip greens, watercress, yellow wax beans, zucchini.

Fruits—none.

Cheese—all cheeses, preferably low fat (no cheese spreads).

Nuts—¼ cup almonds, use for snacks only.

Yogurt—4 oz. plain, may season with cinnamon or other spice.

Bread, bread products, crackers, etc.—none.

Grains—wheat germ.

Fats and oils—butter, soft margarine, vegetable oil spreads, vegetable oils (canola preferable).

Beverages—water, seltzer water and clear broth.

Condiments—salt, pepper, lemon juice, mustard, horseradish, vinegar and all sugar free spices.

Tobacco products—cigarettes and tobacco products should be reduced another 50% during the second week. For example you had cut your cigarettes to 10 a day by the end of the first week, now reduce that 10 to 5 cigarettes per day by the end of the second week.

Sample Menu and Schedule—use only as a guide, eat as many different foods from the above list as you desire

    6am Snack, imperative, must be done every morning
        ¾ cup yogurt while sitting on edge of bed, then lie back and meditate for 3–4 minutes; for exercise, flex fingers, toes, arms and legs ten times each. Then get up and go to the bathroom.
    6:15 Breakfast—omelet
        slice roast beef
        8 oz. glass water
    6:30 Shower, dress and get on with your day.
    8:00 Snack—¼ cup almonds
    9:45 Snack—swiss cheese and pepper strips

11:30 Lunch—vegetable salad with chicken pieces
  seltzer water or 8 oz. glass of water
 2:00 Snack—mung bean sprouts and ¼ cup plain yogurt
 4:15 Snack—radishes and 1" cube cheese
 6:30 Dinner—Super eggplant Parmesan (recipe in back of book)
  asparagus
  wax beans
  salad
  8 oz. glass water
11:00 Snack imperative, must be done every night just before getting into
  bed—¾ cup yogurt

Third Week

Eat only the foods listed.

Fowl—broiled or roasted turkey, chicken or duck. No gravy, filling
  or sauces.

Fish and shellfish—all, but no breading or sauces.

Meats—broiled, roasted or baked beef, veal, pork and lamb. No
  breading, gravies or sauces.

Eggs—any style.

Cereal—No more than 1 serving a day; Oat Bran or non instant
  Oatmeal, add a pat of butter or margarine and/or 1 Tbs. toasted
  wheat germ, sprinkled on top. Absolutely no form of sweetener
  is to be used.

Milk—for cereal and cooking.

Vegetables—alfalfa sprouts, asparagus, bamboo shoots, beet
  greens, broccoli, raw cabbage, cauliflower, celery, chives, collards, cucumber, dandelion greens, eggplant, endive, escarole,
  fennel, green beans, kale, kohlrabi, lettuce, mung bean spouts,
  mushrooms, okra, olives, onions, parsley, sweet peppers, dill
  pickles, pimientos, radishes, swiss chard, tofu, soybean milk,
  spinach, tomatoes, turnips, turnip greens, watercress, yellow
  wax beans, zucchini.

Fruits—only 1 serving per day, watch for any side effects because
  fruit has natural sugar—½ avocado, 1 cup strawberries, 1 cup
  watermelon. Lemon and lime for flavor enhancement.

Cheese—all cheeses, preferably low fat (no cheese spreads).

Nuts—one serving equals a ¼ cup of the following:
  almonds, butternuts, coconut, filberts, hickory, pecans, pistachio and walnuts. Use for snacks only.

Yogurt—plain, may add strawberries or spices.

Bread, bread products, crackers, etc.—1 serving per day; 1 slice
  whole grain bread (½ slice at a time) or 4 whole grain Kavli
  crackers (2 at a time).

Grains and seeds no more than 1 serving a day—wheat germ raw,
  sprouted or cooked, oats, sunflower, sesame, pumpkin, flax-

seed, chia; wheat, mung beans, alfalfa seeds and soy beans are excellent sprouts. (cooked grains—be sure to add a pat of butter).

Fats and oils—butter, soft margarine, vegetable oil spreads, vegetable oils (canola preferable).

Beverages—4 oz. milk per day, water, seltzer water and clear broth.

Condiments—salt, pepper, lemon juice, mustard, horseradish, vinegar and all sugar free spices.

Tobacco products—tobacco usage is to be reduced by 50% again. For example you should be down to 2½ cigarettes per day by the end of the third week.

Sample Menu and Schedule—use only as a guide, eat as many different foods from the above list as you desire. As a general principle you will begin eating less protein and more carbohydrates.

6am Snack, imperative, must be done every morning.
   ¾ cup yogurt while sitting on edge of bed, then lie back and meditate for 3–4 minutes; for exercise, flex fingers, toes, arms and legs ten times each. Then get up and go to the bathroom.

6:15 Breakfast—soft boiled egg(s)
   ½ slice whole grain toast with butter or margarine
   8 oz. glass water

6:30 Shower, dress and get on with your day.

8:00 Snack—¼ cup pistachio nuts

9:45 Snack—¼ cup yogurt with cinnamon

11:30 Lunch—consomme
   ½ slice whole grain bread with butter or margarine
   slices of roast beef and avocado
   Caesar salad without croutons
   8 oz. glass of water or seltzer water

2:00 Snack—1 cup watermelon

4:15 Snack—¼ cup sunflower seeds

6:30 Dinner—roast chicken
   broccoli with lemon juice
   cooked turnips
   spinach salad
   8 oz. glass water

11:00 Snack, imperative, must be done every night just before getting into bed—¾ cup yogurt

Fourth Week

Eat only the foods listed.

Fowl—broiled or roasted turkey, chicken or duck. No gravy, filling or sauces.

Fish and shellfish—all, but no breading or sauces.

Meats—broiled, roasted or baked beef, veal, pork and lamb. No breading, gravies or sauces.

Eggs—any style.

Cereal—No more than 1 serving a day; Oat bran or oatmeal, add a pat of butter or margarine.

Milk—for cereal and cooking.

Vegetables—alfalfa sprouts, asparagus, bamboo shoots, beet greens, broccoli, raw cabbage, cauliflower, celery, chives, collards, cucumber, dandelion greens, eggplant, endive, escarole, fennel, green beans, kale, kohlrabi, lettuce, mung bean spouts, mushrooms, okra, olives, onions, parsley, sweet peppers, dill pickles, pimientos, radishes, swiss chard, tofu, soybean milk, spinach, tomatoes, turnips, turnip greens, watercress, yellow wax beans, zucchini.

Fruits—Eat only one serving per day, watch for any side effects because fruit has natural sugar—½ avocado, ¼ cantaloup, ¼ casaba melon, ½ grapefruit, guava, ½ orange, ½ cup pineapple, 1 cup strawberries, 1 cup watermelon. Lemon and lime for flavor enhancement.

Cheese—all cheeses, preferably low fat. (no cheese spreads)

Nuts—one serving equals a ¼ cup of the following:
almonds, butternuts, coconut, filberts, hickory, pecans, pistachio, walnuts and peanut butter (unsweetened) 1 tablespoon.

Yogurt—plain, may add strawberries or spices or above fruits to it.

Bread, bread products, crackers, etc.—1 serving per day; 1 slice whole grain bread (½ slice at a time) or 4 whole grain Kavli crackers (2 at a time).

Grains and seeds no more than 1 serving a day—wheat germ raw, sprouted or cooked, oats, sunflower, sesame, pumpkin, flaxseed, chia; wheat, mung beans, alfalfa seeds and soy beans are excellent sprouts. (cooked grains—be sure to add a pat of butter).

Fats and oils—butter, soft margarine, vegetable oil spreads, vegetable oils (canola preferable).

Beverages—4 oz. milk per day, water, seltzer water and clear broth.

Condiments—salt, pepper, lemon juice, mustard, horseradish, vinegar and all sugar free spices.

Tobacco products—by the end of the fourth week you should have stopped all tobacco products completely for the rest of your life. Your blood chemistry and subsequently your body chemistry requires it—that's the bottom line.

Sample Menu and Schedule—use only as a guide, eat as many different foods from the above list as you desire. As a general principle you will continue eating less protein and more carbohydrates.

6am Snack, imperative, must be done every morning
¾ cup yogurt while sitting on edge of bed, then lie back and meditate

for 3–4 minutes; for exercise, flex fingers, toes, arms and legs ten
times each. Then get up and go to the bathroom.

6:15 Breakfast—1 cup oat bran cereal with ½ cup milk
  ½ grapefruit
  8 oz. glass water
6:30 Shower, dress and get on with your day.
8:00 Snack—½ cup cottage cheese
9:45 Snack—½ stalk celery filled with peanut butter
11:30 Lunch—opened faced broiled tomato and cheese sandwich (1 slice
  bread) vegetable salad with oil and vinegar
  seltzer water or 8 oz. glass of water
2:00 Snack—raw cauliflower
4:15 Snack—¼ cup walnuts
6:30 Dinner—No-dough zucchini lasagna (recipe in back of book)
  beet greens
  steamed green bean and onions
  8 oz. glass water
11:00 Snack, imperative, must be done every night just before getting into
  bed—¾ cup yogurt

Second Month of the Krimmel Program

Presuming you have subscribed faithfully to the first month's food
ethic you have more than likely enjoyed many positive changes.

Your next step is to *gradually* add some foods of higher carbohydrate concentration and slightly decrease the amount of protein you
eat. You should be watchful for any changes and/or adverse effects
when adding these foods. You must remember that even though we
are all alike in our basic body chemistry, we are all very different in
our individual body chemistry. What may be detrimental to one person may not be to another.

Continue to follow the 4th week plan and add the following foods
to those you are already allowed. Try them in small amounts and not
more than one new food every three days.

Vegetables, these should be eaten in small amounts, ¼ cup, and
  not with bread or fruit—globe artichokes, beets, cooked cabbage, raw carrots, cooked soybeans, winter squash.
Fruits—¼ cup blueberries, ¼ cup boysenberries, ¼ casaba melon, ½
  cup gooseberries, ⅛ honeydew melon, ½ kiwi, 1 medium peach.
Bread, bread products, crackers, etc.—2 whole grain Kavli crackers.
Juices—½ cup only—tomato, V–8, sauerkraut.

If you find yourself losing ground or symptoms returning or you
just don't feel right, cut back on fruits, bread and maybe some higher
percentage carbohydrate vegetables. Remember, do not eat more than
1 slice of bread and no more than one serving of fruit a day. Fruit
and bread should not be eaten together.

Third Month of the Krimmel Program

By this time we suppose you have gained a very large measure of your blood sugar stability. However, rest assured that although you deserve credit for your progress and effort there is still some work to be done and even more gains to be made.

If you haven't been practicing your food ethic 100% or near, there is no magic wand for catching up. You may have to return to the first week and begin over if you feel your progress has not been adequate. If you find it necessary to return to the first week, please discipline yourself this time so you can reap the benefits.

In the third month you will again add some more foods of higher carbohydrate concentration to the foods already allowed in the second month. You will try them in small amounts, one at a time not more often than every third day. Some people will have no problems from these foods and others may not be able to handle some or any of them.

Foods to add:

Vegetables, these vegetables should be eaten in small amounts, ¼ cup, and not with bread or fruit—Jerusalem artichokes, Brussels sprouts, cooked carrots, leeks, lentils, parsnips, peas, split peas, rutabaga.

Fruits—½ cup applesauce, ¼ cup mulberries, medium nectarine, ½ papaya, ¼ cup raspberries, 1 tangerine, 1 clementine.

Juices, ½ cup only—apple, grapefruit, orange.

Desert—fruit, plain gelatin made with allowable fruit and juices. ⟵ See recipes in back of book.

Again, let me repeat, if you find yourself losing ground or your symptoms returning or you just don't feel right, cut back on fruits, bread, juices and maybe some if not all of the higher percentage carbohydrate vegetables you have been eating.

When you have completed the first 3 months of the Krimmel Program, congratulations will be in order. We know that some of the demands the program requires are difficult. It's so hard to control your desires for the sake of a healthy and well controlled body chemistry. But as the months go by you will discover still more and more benefits from your effort. You will be proud of yourself and you will have every right to be.

Two primary things must be continued for the rest of your life if you wish to stay stable:

1) Your time schedule—getting up, eating, exercising and going to bed

2) Your food ethic

Food Ethic For The Rest of Your Life

This section presents your lifetime food guide as to what foods you may eat and those to avoid. Remember, your long term food ethic is high carbohydrate (50–65% of calories), low protein (10–12% of calories) and low fat (20–30% of calories), not high protein. There are foods you may eat in any quantity, foods which may be eaten in small portion infrequently and foods that you must avoid.

Foods You May Eat

- Fish, seafood, fowl, meats—broiled, baked, roasted, sauteed; no breading, gravy or sauce. Sauces and gravies may have MSG, cornstarch and/or white flour. (see "meats to avoid" below)
- Dairy products—eggs, milk, plain yogurt, all cheeses except cheese spreads.
- Soups—those made with allowable foods and no thickening agents, sugar and/or MSG. It is best to make your own. (see recipes in LBS Cookbook)
- Vegetables—those having up to and including 15% carbohydrate content (see list below).
- Fruits—those having up to and including 15% carbohydrate content (see list below).
- Beverages—those having up to and including 15% carbohydrte content (see list below).
- Nuts & Seeds—all, but are high in fat. Eat no more than ¼ cup 2 times a day.
- Cereals—those containing no sugar and dried fruits such as oatmeal, oat bran, shredded wheat, Puffed Kashi, some granolas but may be high in fat. Read labels carefully and know names for different types of sugars (see below).
- Grains—all whole grains, except grits, but in small amounts infrequently.
- Pasta—those made with whole grain flours, artichoke and/or spinach flours, in small amount and infrequently. Beware, many pasta sauces are made with sugar.
- Bread, bread products, crackers, etc—do not eat with gravy, sauce or 15% carbohydrates. Eat ony those made with soya, artichoke, oat, rye and whole grain flours, and little or no sweetener. Have 1 to 3 slices of bread daily and only ½ to 1 slice at a time. Pancakes, waffles, and pizza crust are great made from the above flours. See recipes in back of book and LBS Cookbook.
- Fats and oils—butter, margarine, vegetable oil spreads, vegetable oils (preferably canola).
- Condiments—all, except those containing sugar and/or starch, read labels carefully. Many items contain sugar that you would not suspect, such as ketchup and some mustards.

Listed below are various foods and their percentage of carbohydrate content. Do not eat two items from the 15% list in one meal. Remember, carbohydrates convert to sugar (glucose).

Vegetables

3% to 5% Carbohydrates—no limit on amount or frequency.

bamboo shoots	endive	parsley
beet greens	escarole	peppers, sweet
celery	fennel	pickles, dill & sour
chicory	kale	poke
Chinese cabbage	lettuce	radishes
chives	mushrooms	spinach
collard greens	mustard greens	turnip greens
cucumbers	olives	watercress

6% to 9% Carbohydrates—no limit on amount or frequency.

asparagus	chard	peppers, hot
bamboo shoots	dandelion greens	pimentos
bean sprouts	eggplant	sauerkraut
beans—green & wax	kohlrabi	summer squash
broccoli	okra	tomato
cabbage	onions	turnips
cauliflower	peas, edible pods	zucchini

10% to 14% Carbohydrates—have vegetables from this list only once per day, be watchful of quantity.

artichoke—globe	celeriac	soybeans
beets	chervil	soybean sprouts
Brussels sprouts	leeks	squash, winter
carrots	rutabaga	tomato puree
		water chestnuts

15% + Carbohydrates—Have only a small serving. Do not eat two of these vegetables in the same day or with bread, gravy, or 10% or 15% fruit.

artichoke, Jerusalem	parsnips	split peas
kidney beans	peas	

Vegetables to eat seldom and in very small portion

black eyed peas	lentils	potatoes
corn & corn products	lima beans	sweet potatoes
dried beans & peas	navy beans	yams

Vegetables to avoid

blackbeans	hominy	sweet relish
garbanzos (chickpeas)	sweet pickles	pinto beans

Fruits

It is well recognized that fruit is an important part of your nutritional and aesthetic desires. However, since fruit is very high in natural sugar (simple carbohydrate), some LBS sufferers cannot tolerate any fruit, others can handle a small amount infrequently, while some can tolerate a small amount daily.

Guess who is the only person in the world who can tell how much fruit you are able to eat? You guessed it, only you can determine the frequency and amount of fruit you are able to eat. It will depend on how you feel and function on the day of and/or a day or two after eating fruit. If symptoms return, fruit should be one of the first items consdered to be the cause; therefore eat fruit of lower carbohydrate concentration or eat less fruit or stop eating fruit completely.

No matter what position you take, every once in a while you should consider not eating fruit and drinking juices for a two or three week period and see if your brain clears up (the clouds go away) in how it and you are functioning (less anxiety and/or mood swings). During this period you may also want to cut back or stop eating all starchy foods (breads, pasta, rice, potatoes, corn and other grains).

5% to 9% Carbohydrates—1 cup serving

avocado	guava	strawberries
cantaloupe	loquat	watermelon
grapefruit		

10% to 14% Carbohydrates—½ cup serving

applesauce, unsweetened	gooseberries	orange
apricots, fresh	honeydew melon	papaya
blackberries	kiwi	peach
blueberries	lemon	pineapple
boysenberries	lime	pomegranate
casaba melon	lychee	quince
cranberries, unsweetened	mulberries	raspberries
	muskmelon	tangerines
	nectarines	

15% + Carbohydrates—do not eat daily and eat only a very small portion with caution in mind; do not eat with other fruits or with 15% vegetables or bread.

apples	elderberries	pears
cherries	kumquat	persimmons
coconut, fresh	loganberries	plums
currants, black	mango	youngberries
dewberries	passion fruit	

Fruits to eat seldom and in very small portion

banana	grapes

Fruits to avoid

dates	figs	plantain
dried fruit	fruits canned in syrup	prunes

Beverages:

Healthwise it is recommended that you drink 6 to 8 eight ounce glasses of water a day. The cells in your body need moisture to be healthy. This water is not the water that is in any other beverage, it is plain water.

Even though herb teas have no caffeine, you should be wary of them because they may have a natural substance which is detrimental and also they may put you back in the habit of desiring or even drinking regular tea and coffee.

0% to 4% Carbohydrates
 clear broth   seltzer water   water
 herb tea

5% to 9% Carbohydrates—½ cup per day
 milk   tomato juice   vegetable juice
 sauerkraut juice

10% to 14% Carbohydrates—½ cup per day
 apple juice   grapefruit juice
 blackberry juice orange juice   pomegranate juice
 carrot juice   tangerine juice

15% + Carbohydrates—½ cup per day
 apricot nectar   pear nectar   raspberry juice
 loganberry juice pineapple juice

Beverages to avoid

alcohol	grape juice	soft drinks
cocoa	ovaltine	strong tea
coffee	papaya juice	excessive amounts of
colas	postum	any fruit or
chocolate	prune juice	vegetable juice.

Other Foods To Avoid—items that have any type of sugar and/or artificial sweetener, cornstarch or MSG added.

Breads, bread products and crackers—made with white flour and/or sugar

bread	pancakes	pretzels
crackers	pizza	waffles
matzo		

Pasta—all made from white flour

lasagne	manicotti	ravioli
macaroni	noodles	spaghetti
noodles		

Meats—all lunch meats and cold cuts; usually have some form of sugar and fillers, read labels carefully.

bacon	ham	sausage
canned meats	hot dogs	scrapple
cold cuts	lunch meats	

Snack food

| corn chips | popcorn | potato chips |

Desserts—anything made with white flour and/or sugar

cake	ice cream	pie
cookies	Jello-O	puddings
custards	pastry	

Sweets

| candy | jam | molasses |
| caramel | jelly | sugar |

chewing gum   malt   syrup
honey   marmalade

Following are various names for sugar; all should be avoided:

Barley malt	Galactose	Mannose
Black Strap Molasses	Glucose	Maple syrup
Cane syrup	Glycerin	Molasses
Caramel	Hexitol	Natural sweeteners
Caramel coloring	Honey	Rice syrup
Corn syrup	Lactose	Simple syrup
Corn syrup solids	Levulose	Sorbitol
Dextrin	Licorice	Sorghum
Dextrose	Malt	Sucrose
Disaccharide	Maltose	Syrup
Fructose	Mannitol	Xylitol

On some product labels you won't find sugar per se listed on the ingredient list. Labeling laws require only added ingredients to be listed not ingredients that are in the product naturally. A good example is milk. Milk is usually thought of as a protein food whereas it actually has more carbohydrate than protein. Much of the carbohydrate is in the form of lactose, a sugar. That is why milk is limited in the Krimmel Program.

Products With No Added Sugar

Following are a few products that have no added sugar. It is very important to get into the habit of reading the ingredient list on all products. Manufacturers seem to have a habit of changing ingredients in their products. A product that does not have sugar at one time may later have it and vice versa.

Yogurt—Dannon, plain
Cottage cheese—Breakstone, regular
Applesauce—Motts Natural Style
    Musselmans Natural Style
    Lucky Leaf Old Fashioned Natural
    Seneca 100% Natural
Pineapple—Dole, in its own juice
    3 Diamonds, in its own juice
    Empress, in its own juice
Peanut butter—Crazy Richard
    Smuckers' Natural
    Old Dominion
    Peter Pan—No sugar added
Crackers—Wasa Brod, whole rye
    Kavli, Norwegian flatbread thin
Cereal—Oat Bran
    Quacker Puffed Rice and Wheat
    Shredded Wheat

Quaker Oats
Cream of Wheat
Jams & jellies—made with only fruit but high in natural sugar
Polaner All Fruit
Sorrell Ridge
Smuckers'—Simply Fruit
Strawberries—Ideal, frozen in a bag
Peaches—Ideal, frozen in a bag
Tomato sauce—Contadina Italian style
Acme
Spaghetti sauce—Classico Di Napoli
Hunt's Homestyle
Aunt Millie's Old Fashioned Italian style
Juices—all high in natural sugar
Dole Pure & Light
Apple & Eve
Nice & Natural
After the Fall
Most Apple juices
V-8

Ideas For Snacks

The primary purpose of snacks is to supply a constant, even supply of energy to the body. The snacks prevent a severe dip of blood sugar between meals. The snacks act as a bridge of energy between meals. For example if a very early breakfast is eaten, 2 snacks may be needed before lunch. Likewise, if a late dinner is planned, 2 or more afternoon snacks may be needed. Most people need to eat every 1½ to 2 hours in order to keep their blood sugar stable. After being on the progrram for awhile, you will probably discover and develop your best eating patterns. This is a personal learning process.

Following are some enjoyable snacks:

- Celery with peanut butter.
- Peanut butter on thin slices of apple.
- Whole rye crackers with unsweetened peanut butter.
- Cheddar cheese and ½ sour apple.
- ½ cup plain yogurt with 2 Tbs. applesauce and ½ tsp. cinnamon mixed.
- ½ cup plain yogurt mixed with fresh chopped fruit.
- Handful of nuts—almonds, peanuts, brazil, butternuts, pumpkin or squash seeds, black walnuts and pecans.
- Hard boiled egg.
- Fresh fruit—cherries, ½ grapefruit, ½ orange, tangerine, pear, ½ cup pineapple, strawberries, ½ sour apple, ¼ cantaloupe or peach.
- ¾ cup cottage cheese with 3 Tbs. crushed pineapple.
- Carrot and celery sticks.
- Raw broccoli, cauliflower, pepper strips.

See our Low Blood Sugar Cookbook for additional snacks.

Learn How Your Body Reacts to Various Foods

After you have eaten only the allowable foods for 3 months you will find that your desire for sweets has greatly diminished. When you feel you have become very stable you might want to try something with sugar in it when you are at a party, but you dare eat only a very small portion—*don't pig out!* Let me warn you of a couple of things, sweets will taste exceptionally sweet now and even though you do not seem to be affected by the sweets immediately, don't think you can eat all you want or you will be right back where you started, square one, the first week.

If you cheat by eating foods not allowed or allowed foods to which you react or by using stimulants, you are going to pay, usually within 72 hours, the time period needed by the body to throw off any intruders. This has been a general observation, try it on yourself. The most important point is—learn to observe and interpret your own body's actions and reactions to the substances with which it comes in contact. For example, if Ed. eats macaroni or spaghetti, the next day he suffers a collection of side effects such as tiredness, blurred vision, sneezing, mood swings, etc. This may last for 2 to 3 days. In effect, what we are trying to show you is that your body has a language through which it sends messages. The messages are sent by the side effects from your cheating or, to put it positively, you will feel great when your body is being given the substances which are most compatible to it.

Special Note

You must be alert to two factors in relation to your food ethic:

1. Eat quality foodstuffs for a quality energy supply which will result in a quality life style and body chemistry. This is not the pursuit of the best tasting—though it certainly isn't blah—or the most expensive or exotic food—but the best quality food chemistry which will lead to a true blue flame in the fires of your body's chemistry. Think true blue flame when selecting foods to eat.

2. Don't overeat—eat just enough to maintain a constant quality supply of energy to your brain and body. You have grown up in a society which teaches more means better—well, you must think less is best. The best quality and the least you can get by with. Don't smother your blue flame by pouring too much on it—even though the foodstuffs are of the best quality. Too much of anything, even the best of something can be injurious. Learn to live on the edge of having just enough food each time you eat, not too much—think blue flame and never fall into the trap of eating too much at any time—meal or snack. Remember, it's possible if you eat too much you'll feel rotten—if you eat too little you'll feel rotten—that's the way it is.

The 90 Days No Excuse Menu

This 90 day menu is for those who are unable, for one or more reasons, to prepare a cooked variety of foods. This is a no bells, no whistles and no frills menu to follow for 90 days. You may not get any esthetic enrichment but your body chemistry will be fined tuned.

6am Snack, imperative, must be done every morning
¾ cup plain, low fat yogurt while sitting on edge of bed, then lie back and meditate for 3–4 minutes; for exercise, flex fingers, toes, arms and legs ten times each. Then get up and go to the bathroom.

6:15 Breakfast—eggs, shredded wheat or unsweetened granola
¼–½ cup low fat milk
½ grapefruit or ½ orange beginning fourth week
8 oz. glass water

6:30 Shower, dress and get on with your day.

8:00 Snack—½ cup low fat cottage cheese

9:45 Snack—½ stalk celery filled with 1 Tbs. unsweetened peanut butter

11:30 Lunch—choice of hard boiled eggs, cold roast beef, cheese or cold chicken or turkey (don't use Deli meats)
vegetables, raw or cooked, two or more of the following:

alfalfa sprouts	carrots	olives
asparagus	cauliflower	peppers
beans, green & wax	celery	radishes
bean sprouts	cucumber	spinach
broccoli	lettuce	tomato
cabbage	mushrooms	tofu
		zucchini

seltzer water or 8 oz. glass of water

2:00 Snack—handful of various seeds and nuts

4:15 Snack—raw vegetable with 1" cube cheese

6:30 Dinner—choice of tuna, sardines, cold chicken or turkey, roast beef (don't use Deli meats)
vegetables, raw or cooked, two or more of the following:

alfalfa sprouts	carrots	olives
asparagus	cauliflower	peppers
beans, green & wax	celery	radishes
bean sprouts	cucumber	spinach
broccoli	lettuce	tomato
cabbage	mushrooms	tofu
		zucchini

8 oz. glass of water

11:00 Snack, imperative, must be done every night just before getting into bed—¾ cup plain, low fat yogurt

Beginning the third week you may have 1 slice of whole grain bread (½ slice at a time) or 4 whole grain Kavli crackers (2 at a time) daily.

EXERCISE

For stabilizing your body chemistry exercise plays as important a role as food—and in some respects more of one. It is the second dimension we are discussing—but it's equal to the first dimension discussed—food ehtic. You must begin to include it in your everyday schedule—just as you include food and water.

What Is Exercise?

Exercise is the regular active use of the body in order to make it stronger and healthier. This activity should increase your heart rate for several minutes.

Why Exercise?

Oxygen is the most important substance required by the body. You can live days without food and water but only 5 minutes without oxygen. The amount of oxygen you take in is in direct proportion to the amount of physical activity you do.

Exercise is one of the vital means of building a wall of resistance between you and degenerative conditions—LBS being one of these degenerative conditions. Once you have a degenerative condition, exercise is one of the vital means of overcoming or controlling the condition.

What Does Exercise Do?

Exercise makes us stronger and healthier by improving the oxygen intake and delivery to our body. When we exercise we breathe deeper and faster thereby increasing our lung capacity. Exercise also makes the heart pump (beat) stronger and faster which strengthens the heart muscle. Our major blood vessels enlarge due to the increased rate and amount of blood being pumped through them. All of this leads to an improved ability to use oxygen and an increased ability to deliver nutrients to each and every cell by our improved circulatory system, improved digestion, absorption, metabolism, and the improved elimination of our waste products.

Philosophy of Exercise

Exercise is very personal, what is suited to one person may be totally unsuited to another—for a variety of reasons. For starters, you must take a very close look at where you are now in relation to your physical well-being and where you wish to go. After a clear picture is seen of the now and then—you can begin charting a course on how to get there and by what stages. You must decide on the time of day and the type and degree of exercise. Each area of the program must remain interesting to you and goal oriented.

You should not feel you have to do the same activities for exercise every day. If you were on vacation at the seashore and spent the majority of your time in the ocean fighting the waves and briskly walking the beach, that would be your exercise.

Another factor of importance and probably of the highest priority is that you must make sure the exercise program you choose is fun and interesting to you. Avoid fad or cosmetic type exercises and programs. It has been established scientifically that people who participate in exercises and activities that are not pleasurable to them do themselves more harm than good. Regardless of scientific findings, if you were to just sit and ponder the mood that is generated when participating in activities that are not to your liking you will gradually see the point and importance of this issue. The value of exercise is in direct proportion to how your body's mechanisms are responding to the mood which is being created during the given activity.

Perhaps an example will bring this subtle but vital point into focus. Take an introverted person who somehow decides jogging is good for him. The majority of jogging is done on a public thoroughfare and tends to be an exhibitionist activity, which would generally be distressing to an introverted personality. From a premise of conjecture we can visualize our individual's body chemistry and its mechanism being in a defensive position rather than an offensive position. An exaggeration of this example would be the person jogging with clenched fist in contrast to loose open hands. Very simply, you want to pursue happy, relaxed, pleasant, and stimulating activities, not begrudging ones.

Before you begin exercising you should be checked by your doctor.

Types of Exercise

There are 3 primary types of exercise:

   1. Warm-up   2. Conditioning   3. Circulatory

Warm-up exercises stretch and limber up the muscles and increase the heart and lung action, thereby preparing the body for greater exertion and reducing the possibility of unnecessary strain. An excellent time to do some stretching and arm and leg bending, particularly for LBS people, is before getting out of bed. A two minute session is highly recommended—watch a baby or a cat when they awaken, they instinctively stretch and bend their extremities.

Examples of warm-up exercises:

Bending and stretching	Knee bends
Bending side to side	Knee lifts

Conditioning exercises are to tone up major muscles such as the abdomen, back, legs, arms, etc.

Examples of conditioning exercises:

Knee push ups	Sit ups	Hiking
Touching toes	Bicycling	Skating

Circulatory exercises produce contraction of large muscle groups for relatively longer periods than conditioning to stimulate and strengthen the circulatory and respiratory system.

Examples of circulatory exercises:

Brisk walk	Bicycling	Swimming
Jumping rope	Tennis—singles	Cross-country skiing

Things to Remember When Exercising

When is it best for you to exercise? Some people find that when they first get up is best, but for LBS people this may be the least favorable time because they may deplete their energy too much or too quickly. Decide when you feel the best during the day and that would perhaps be the most ideal time to exercise.

- Don't "bankrupt" yourself of your energy reserve—never do more exercise and use more energy than you can afford to spend at your level of blood sugar stability.
- It is preferable that you wait for at least an hour after you eat before doing any strenuous activity so it doesn't interfere with your digestion.
- If you have not been doing any type of exercise, start out slowly by going for short brisk walks. Gradually increase the briskness and distance. LBS people should not over exert themselves when beginning an exercise program.
- When your exercise time becomes more strenuous and longer, have an apple or something else with you to eat in case you feel the need for food.
- Do activities that are enjoyable to you, your activities can change with the seasons—swimming in summer; ice skating or cross country skiing or sledding in the winter; biking or hiking in the fall and spring. Of course brisk walking can be done almost anytime and anywhere. Doing yard or garden work or hard housework (scrubbing) for a couple of hours is also good.

Pulse Taking

In order for exercise to be effective and to produce the desired results, your pulse rate must increase to a certain point. Exercise should be done for 20 to 30 minutes at a time depending on blood sugar stability, at least three to four times a week. See the chart below for what your pulse rate should increase to during your exercise.

PULSE RATE DURING EXERCISE			
AGE	*PULSE RATE*	*AGE*	*PULSE RATE*
20	120–150 beats per minute	50	102–127 beats per minute
25	117–146 beats per minute	55	99–123 beats per minute
30	114–142 beats per minute	60	96–120 beats per minute
35	111–138 beats per minute	65	93–116 beats per minute
40	108–135 beats per minute	70	90–113 beats per minute
45	105–131 beats per minute		

Source: U.S. Department of Health and Human Services

To take your pulse, put the 3 middle fingers of your right hand on the under side of your left wrist below your thumb. Count the beats for 30 seconds and multiply by 2 for how many beats per minute.

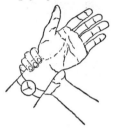

Cold Extremities

Many LBS people have cold hands and feet even when the rest of their body is warm. For these people it is a good idea to exercise their fingers and toes and rub them gently. This stimulates circulation to the fingers and toes and will help warm them. The increased circulation brings more oxygen to the area to be burned as fuel to make heat.

Summary

In summary, exercise should be an activity that you enjoy doing, which increases your pulse rate and is done at least 3 to 4 times a week in pleasing surroundings. The exercise should improve muscle tone, digestion, metabolism and elimination as well as supplying sufficient oxygen to each and every cell to help insure efficient functioning. The importance of exercise cannot be overstated. Your LBS program is not complete until you have included exercise. However, if exercise has been difficult to maintain because of pain, you may need to go into it very slowly and gently, but regularly. Going out for a short stroll is a beginning. Remember you are not alone on your journey. See you on the path!

FUN AND LAUGHTER

In recent years there has been much written about the benefits of laughter. However, there are very few scientific studies in this area. But the benefits of laughter have been known of for centuries.

The Bible tells us in Proverbs 17:22, "A merry heart doeth good like a medicine; but a broken spirit drieth the bones."

Therapeutic Value of Fun and Laughter

Laughter increases the heart rate and breathing, which leads to an increased intake of oxygen. It also provides another benefit, "internal massaging." The diaphragm moves greatly during laughter, causing a massage-like effect, which increases circulation in nearby organs, helping them to function more efficiently.

Laughter also stimulates the brain to produce catecholamines, which may help release natural pain killers known as endorphins. There are accounts of pepole who had been in pain being able to get a couple of hours of good, pain-free sleep after some hearty laughter.

Fun and laughter help relieve stress and tension, which releases you from your physical and psychological bonds. This is very beneficial to a LBS sufferer.

Some research has established that negative moods generate negative chemical changes in the body. Dare we assume that positive emotions (fun and laughter) generate positive chemical changes? If this is so, it surely is another valuable contribution in stabilizing your blood sugar.

Where and How to Find Fun and Laughter

Do you play for fun, laughter and enjoyment or do you play to see who is the best and who can win? It doesn't require very keen powers of observation to observe that most of the activities in the U.S. culture are geared to the excitement of winning and seeing who is the best. Much of this has come about by incorporating most activities into formal events, where winning is the goal and patrons can be charged for attending the events.

Whatever happened to playing a game for fun and comradery? When was the last time you played cards, ball, tennis or whatever just for the fun of it, not caring who won?

We are talking about fun, not excitement. Some excitement is fun. But there is excitement that is more anxiety-producing than fun-producing. For instance a race track in contrast to an amusement park.

Having fun usually involves an activity with 2 or more people and the avoidance of over regulation. Playing volley ball strictly by the rules is not nearly as much fun as just playing for the sake of playing. This was brought home to us recently when a group of adults and children were playing volley ball by very loose rules. The children said they disliked volley ball at school but really liked playing it with us and it was the best fun they ever had. This holds true to many other activities as well—so be careful of sticking strictly to the rules.

Also be aware of "artificial fun" created through alcohol and its environment.

Some of the places we have found to be most fun-producing are:

Picnics—where there are activities such as baseball, volley ball, horseshoes, frisbees and other freeflowing activities, where winning is not the main concern but fun is.

Beach—where you have the freedom to run, swim, yell and just plain relax.

Amusement parks—there you can vent your emotions on the rides without feeling conspicuous.

Family or friends get together—where good food and conversation is very relaxing.

Hiking and/or camping groups—fellowship of people with the same types of interests.

Bicycle club—exercise and fresh air lend to fun and laughter.

SLEEP, REST AND RELAXATION

The proper sleep, rest and relaxation are as important as the proper food and exercise in helping to stabilize your blood sugar.

Stress is a natural and common dimension of our daily life. The ultimate aim is to control stress so it does not become distress. Sleep, rest and relaxation are the ways the body keeps stress under control. Each of these should be looked upon as an art and the individual should look to improve upon them through a continuous and conscious effort. The ultimate goal is to find a happy balance between sleep, rest, relaxation and stress. Let's deal with each one of them individually.

Sleep

The main purpose of sleep seems to be restorative. All functions of the body are slowed down, except for persipration which increases. This slowed down period gives our systems a chance to rest so they will be able to function efficiently during the next awake period. Perspiration increases to help get rid of waste products while we are sleeping.

The amount and quality of sleep tend to vary according to the age of individuals. Babies require 14 hours of sleep, young adults 8 hours and senior aged persons 5 to 6 hours. Regardless of age, there are always those individuals, such as Napoleon who slept only a couple of hours during the night, however, he would take cat naps during the day.

From having dealt with many LBS persons we find the following generalities to be true:

LBS people tend to be nocturnal people.

LBS people tend to have some type of sleep difficulty such as—going to sleep, waking up during the night, sleeping too deeply, not refreshed when waking up, unable to wake up on time, erratic sleeping hours.

Each individual should strive to determine how much sleep he needs to feel refreshed upon awakening. Too much sleep is just as apt to make you feel sluggish as too little. Go to bed at the same time every night, after eating your snack. The first morning get up after having slept the longest time you think you need, after a few mornings get up ½-hour earlier and keep getting up ½-hour earlier every few days until you have reached what you feel is the least amount of sleep time needed. Keep a record of how you have felt when getting up at these various times and see what amount of sleep gave you the best feeling. Also keep in mind how you felt during the rest of the day when getting up at the various times. After you have determined your adequate hours of sleep do not change your getting up time, even on your days off or vacation. When you want more or less sleep change your hour of going to bed. It is important to standardize your sleeping hours but if they must change, better to change the hour of going to bed if possible rather than the hour of getting up.

We have found an ideal time range for getting up for many LBS persons to be 5:30 a.m. to 7 a.m. There are some who seem to function best from 7 p.m. to 6 a.m. and therefore should sleep during the day—that's great if their lifestyle permits it.

For more information on sleep aides see Snacks Before Going To Bed and Getting Up The Same Time Every Day in the section, "Ideas For Fine Tuning."

Rest

Rest is the mind's and body's freedom from activity. It has been shown to be very beneficial to take a 15-to-30 minute nap after lunch every day. This has two effects—your food has a chance to begin to digest in a relaxed atmosphere and your body can recharge itself and conseve energy for the afternoon's activities. If unable to take a nap, then lie down or put your feet up with a good book or soothing music. Also, disconnect the phone if possible and put up a DO NOT DIS-TURB sign with time available indicated on it.

For LBS sufferers, periodic breaks or rests are invaluable, but don't use them as substitutes for snacks. Also, try to take your rests and breaks at the same time every day so your body has a normal routine. Be alert, often when feeling tired you need a snack, not a nap, to give you a pick up in energy.

A short nap can prove invaluable before major events such as business meetings, social gatherings and trips. Even the enjoyment of going out to dinner and a movie can be increased by taking a short cat nap beforehand.

Relaxation

Relaxation is important and helpful to counterbalance stress and tension. There are various ways to relax, depending on what your normal daily activities are. To someone in an office all day, gardening may be very relaxing. It probably wouldn't do much for a farmer.

Some general suggestions for capturing the mood and benefits of relaxation are, getting out of the immediate work environment, taking a short walk, sitting back and shutting off all interruptions, doing something new and novel, or tinkering. Relaxation means something different to everyone. The ideal is finding something that reduces stress and tension and makes you feel productive and worthwhile, other than your normal major involvements. We know one person who for relaxation and enjoyment washes dishes at home and fixes bicycles for the children in the neighborhood.

Chapter 5

SETTING THE STAGE FOR MAINTAINING YOUR BLOOD SUGAR

Now that you have a clear idea of what low blood sugar is and what the Krimmel Program is, this section will give you some additional aides in the art of staging and maintaining your blood sugar at the proper level.

FRAME OF MIND

It's a good idea for everyone to acquire and maintain a positive frame of mind, but for a person trying to combat low blood sugar, it's essential. Getting and keeping a proper outlook may also be the most difficult part of your recovery—because it is often the low blood sugar you are trying to combat that leads to negative thoughts and actions.

But it can be done. That's why we have written this book. It isn't easy. But it can be done. And there is no question it is worth the effort.

Suggestions for acquiring and maintaining a positive frame of mind:

- Supply your brain with a constant supply of its primary fuel of blood sugar. In order for your brain to function efficiently and positively it must have an adequate supply of blood sugar, which comes from eating the proper foods. And the supply must be delivered at the appropriate times.

- Simplify your overall lifestyle. You must endeavor to get as much stress and as many negative intrusions out of your life as possible. Learn to work toward solutions rather than repeating (physically and verbally) the problems. For example:
  - Keep your home and auto well maintained so you will get pleasure from them rather than aggravation.
  - Live within your income.

- Put on paper your short and long-term goals for life, and work toward these goals.
- Make slow methodical decisions, not hasty ones. Try not to act rashly, when your blood sugar may be low.

- Try to use the following suggestions daily:
  - Look at the bottle as half full, rather than as half empty. Look at every situation for its positive aspects rather than the negative ones.
  - Look at what you are gaining, not what you are giving up. In following the food-ethic, concentrate on how great you feel. No headaches. More dependable energy. No mood swings. Don't keep thinking about what "sweets" you are being "denied."
  - Accentuate the positive, eliminate the negative. For example, when it's raining, see it for the good that is being supplied by nature, not as a dark cloudy day. Don't allow the words of the weatherman to affect you.

- Develop a mental atitude for living and enjoying life one day at a time. Follow the "Krimmel Program" the best you can every day. The success of today has much to do with your actions of yesterday, just as today's actions will have an influence on how you feel and what you accomplish tomorrow. For a LBS sufferer it is often a trade-off of instant gratification for long-term stability and enjoyment. As we often tell the people we work with: *"Don't let the tip of your tongue rule your body's chemistry and your free will."* Of course we remind them that the "tip of your tongue" is where your sweet taste buds live.

- The next time you feel like having some junk food maybe the following concepts can be helpful.
  - Pain and discomfort—If you suffer consequences after eating some of the "no-no" foods, you will have to face the truth that this substance is a poison to you. It is tarnishing your body, your "Temple."
  - Self-discipline—You must be mature about this and not rationalize or let others trap you into eating things that are harmful to your body chemistry.
  - Knowledge—Knowing your body chemistry and nutrition and how they interact is of utmost importance.

EBB AND FLOW

Classically the concept of ebb and flow relates to the ocean tide. The water comes in and goes out, comes in and goes out, in and out. Each time the water comes in onto the beach a little farther with a rising tide. So it often is with a low blood sugar sufferer. You make progress and then you slip back a little, you make a little more progress and again you slip back a little. But bear in mind that just as the tide rises to its ultimate level so you, too, will reach your ultimate level of blood-sugar stability, providing you continue your program with a conscientious effort.

Another thing you must be aware of is that there will be times that even though you are following the program faithfully your symptoms will return for no obvious reasons. The best we can tell you is that the longer you follow the program the less often these relapses will occur. If and when they do occur you must remember not to let them demoralize you. Stick with your program. Understand clearly that they will pass.

We do suggest that you try to review the things that have occurred in your life in the past 2 or 3 days. Things to be especially aware of are unusual stress, exposure to chemical substances (paint, perfumes, auto and industrial emissions, etc.) deviations of food program (restaurants) and illnesses (virus, colds, etc.).

One last dimension about the ebb and flow of your body chemistry that needs to be remembered is that the more pure it becomes, the more sensitive it becomes. This tends to happen only in the first few months of the program. This is similar to your having been exposed to a negative odor for a long time. You don't notice it very much. However, go into the clean, pure air for a short time and when you return, the negative odor seems extremely offensive. So it appears to be with the body's chemistry in relation to low blood sugar. While you were consistently eating fast-acting (refined) carbohydrates your side effects were more or less standardized. Your body was used to being abused. Then you left the fast-acting carbohydrates and went to the pure, slow-acting carbohydrates—and felt better. If you return to the refined carbohydrates your side effects will tend to be much more pronounced, just like the odor was much more pronounced— because your body has learned what it is to function properly!

PILOT-COPILOT RELATIONSHIP— GETTING THROUGH THE CLOUDS

Visualize yourself and another person in the cockpit of a plane. The copilot is a support person for the pilot. So it is with a low blood sugar sufferer, he needs a copilot to support him when he can't navigate properly. The copilot must be:

- Knowledgeable of, or willing to learn low blood sugar concepts.
- Available.
- Interested.
- Compassionate.
- Mature, and willing not to have his feelings hurt (putting his ego aside). When the LBS sufferer loses control and yells at the copilot or does anything derogatory, the important thing is not to take the incident personally—it's not the individual acting this way, it's the LBS crushing his brain.
- Willing to dominate when necessary.

It may be desirable or necessary to enlist more than one copilot. You may want or need more than one copilot in one setting or one copilot for each setting. For example:

- At home all of the family members could possibly be copilots.
- At work maybe only one person would be necessary.

In the final analysis much of this depends on the severity of the low blood sugar and your lifestyle.

Why is a Pilot-Copilot Relationship Necessary?

The copilot must support the low blood sugar sufferer (pilot) when his blood sugar is low because his brain can't function efficiently. The LBS person knows something is wrong but can't correct it because of poor brain functioning. The copilot (support person) must remind him to eat—or even go so far as to hand him the food and maybe put it in his mouth. This might sound ridiculous, but some LBS victims really need this degree of assistance, especially in the beginning of the program until they become somewhat stabilized and they are able to function more efficiently. In our case whenever I would become verbally hostile my wife would actually shove pieces of cheese or other food into my mouth and then leave the room. Within a few moments lo and behold I would feel a positive transition coming about. The fact that this transition occurs is still surprising to us— but very real.

You must remember that it is the brain that enables us to maintain our functions and if the brain is not getting adequate glucose for energy there are going to be deficiencies in its performance.

Here is an analogy to show the point: Dare we expect a blind person to be able to fix a tear in a fine garment? Then why should we expect the LBS sufferer to be able to remember to eat a snack when his blood sugar is low? If his blood sugar was stable, he wouldn't need the snack.

The copilot must be aware of the signs that indicate the blood sugar is falling, and the circumstances that bring the problem on. Following are a few:

- How long has it been since last eating? A LBS victim usually needs to eat every 1½ to 2 hours.
- A vague look in the eyes.
- Falling asleep during the day.
- Irritable for no obvious reason.
- Can't concentrate.

Bear in mind that no two LBS persons are identical and therefore the signs of falling blood sugar vary with each individual. The copilot must become very familiar with his pilot's particular side effects in order to be able to help effectively.

Besides eating on time, the LBS victim at times needs support in eating the proper types of foods. Staying away from all the so-called "goodies" (alcohol, tobacco, sweets, caffeine) of this culture can be torturous when everyone else seems to be "enjoying" them. This is a perfect example of the vital role a copilot can play by encouraging the LBS person to follow his proper food ethic.

The copilot should try to remember as much as possible of the progress the LBS person has made in his recovery. There will be times when this information will be very valuable, in keeping the pilot on course.

Some examples:

- The LBS person is in a negative mood and complains that they haven't made any progress. The copilot can respond: "Are you still having severe headaches, trouble sleeping, blurred vision, etc.?" (of course the questions must be related to the LBS person's individual symptoms)
- The LBS person will say "I am tired of this diet, what good does it do me anyway?" Again the copilot can review the progress made by the LBS person, pointing out that it has been a long time since such and such has happened.
- The LBS person states, "This candy or coffee won't affect me." Again the copilot reviews the progress made and can perhaps remind the LBS sufferer that he growled at the cat the last time he had candy or coffee.

One of the most valuable things we have found to help us understand many of the complaints expressed by low blood sugar victims is a saying from a dear friend of ours: "When a person complains, you must remember that all he or she is really saying and asking is, 'please help me'."

It becomes an enjoyable and rewarding experience for the pilot and copilot to sit down together periodically and review the progress made by their combined efforts. Eventually as the pilot's blood sugar stabilizes and his symptoms lessen, the copilot's role will become greatly diminished, but never forgotten.

How Do You Find Someone at Work to Be Your Copilot?

How do you find someone at work to be supportive and helpful? First of all you must decide who you would be comfortable having help you. Do you want the office clown, the office grouch, the office know-it-all or Miss Nicey-Nice? I doubt you want any of these, you want someone who is dependable, mature and discreet.

You may ask, why should anyone be interested in helping me? Did you ever see anyone helping a diabetic, someone in a wheelchair or someone with a broken arm? Sure you have and no one makes it a big deal, they just help. You are just another human being with a need, reach out and recruit the right person to help you. Thank goodness the Creator in his ultimate wisdom created all types of personalities including the type that needs you to need him. The magic words are—"Will You Please Help Me, I Need You?"

When asking for help you can say that you need help similar to that which a diabetic often needs. You need to be reminded to eat every 1½ to 2 hours, to eat the correct foods and to avoid stimulants (caffeine, alcohol and tobacco). Make sure you explain to your support person that the reason you need to be reminded is that your brain runs low on energy and your memory for eating shuts down unless you eat frequently. Also you may need his encouragement to stay away from sweets, coffee and cigarettes, particularly at coffee break time. Explain that once you become stabilized you more than likely won't need him as regularly if at all.

The ideal is to have your support person do some reading about hypoglycemia. Who knows, his working with you may be the inducement he needs to improve his own body chemistry.

If your work situation permits, you may not need to recruit anyone at work. You could possibly have your spouse, parent, or other call you at work at prearranged times to remind you to eat. My wife used to call me at the real estate office and check to see if I had eaten.

Here are four additional options that may spark some additional thoughts on your part:

1. Contract with a telephone answering service to call you at specified times to remind you to eat.
2. Use a telephone beeper service so you can be reached anywhere when it is time for you to eat.
3. Contract with a local restaurant or the company cafeteria to deliver you small food parcels at specified times.
4. Wear an alarm wrist watch preset for specified times to alert you to eat.

We are not trying to overwhelm you in our suggesting these supportive aides. You will wean away from all this support once you are stabilized and can understand the messages your body is sending you. Some of the messages my body sends me when I need to eat are:

Sneezing	Drowsiness	Yawning
Visual disturbances	Mood swings	Use of four letter
Headaches	Lack of concentration	words

More than likely you will be able to understand your body's language after being on the Krimmel Program for 2 to 6 months.

GETTING ENOUGH INFORMATION

It is extremely important that you begin developing a wider spectrum of information which will allow you to gain greater insights into the low blood sugar condition. The foremost means for accomplishing this is to realize that LBS is a dimension of your overall body chemistry and has a direct relationship to the food chemistry you eat. Subsequently it is imperative that you learn more about body chemistry and food chemistry and how they interact with each other.

The most popular way of gaining information in the western world is through reading (that's how we got you inside our book in the first place). Besides reading, talking with other people who have LBS is helpful. Don't worry about how you find them, they will come from under rocks, from behind trees and out of the woodwork! You'll see! So your first step is to learn enough about LBS to help yourself and then you will recognize others who also have the condition.

The LBS mending process requires you to collect and use information particular to yourself and your condition. You have to collect as much information as possible about LBS, and then be like a jeweler setting fine stones in how you use the information relative to your situation and body chemistry. Perhaps for the first time in your recent past or your whole life, you will be dealing with information which has a specific relationship to your problems.

Every LBS person should be particularly alert and watchful for all LBS information and also for any and all food and body chemistry information. One never knows what new piece of information will give him a large chunk of insight.

To give you an idea of how valuable an additional piece of information can be, let me tell you about a part of the brain called the neocortex. One day I was doing some casual reading and quite by chance I read the following concept in a book by Dr. Lendon Smith. *"When the blood sugar drops from the overproduction of insulin following the ingestion of refined sugar or a food allergen, the part of the brain that is responsible for self-control, the neocortex, is unable to function. The circuits that say 'I'm a nice person; you're a nice person' are simply nonenergized, and lower, more animal responses take over. Selfish, aggressive, antisocial attitudes predominate . . . The part of the brain that has conscious control (the conscience) over the lusts of the flesh is the neocortex, and the neocortex is the first to become nonoperative when the blood sugar falls. ('I ate one piece of candy and soon the whole box was gone.')"*

When I first read this concept, my emotional response was so intense and I was so elated because the concept gave me the insight into why so many hypoglycemics function the way they do. I really found out what Socrates meant when he said, "Knowledge will bring you joy."

Just pause and contemplate the importance of this concept. Here is a piece of information that is the key to understanding why so many LBS individuals are not able to control their behavior when their blood sugar is dipping. In other words if your blood sugar is dipping, the cells in the neocortex will begin shutting down from lack of energy and subsequently that station in your brain which is responsible for maintaining self-control has its lights going out. If this circumstance persists, you will be unable to control what you eat or how you behave emotionally along with a multitude of other things. So when you feel like the world and your brain are falling apart and/ or you begin screaming, ranting and raving, try your darnedest to eat some food to give the neocortex the energy it needs to give you back your self control. Unfortunately you need to use your brain, which is shutting down, to help you remember to eat and this is near impossible, so the best thing is for your copilot to give you the food.

In my opinion this is a good example for showing why you should continue getting more information as well as keeping your blood sugar stable. I hope you feel the same way.

Remember, you are the one who lives inside your body and it's what, how much and how often you feed your body chemistry that controls how you feel and function. If getting more information improves the quality of your life it's a great bargain. After all where are you going to move after your body is worn out?

Limit What Type of Information You Get

There are times when you should consider limiting the type of information you get and how much effort is expressed in getting it. A perfect example is taking the glucose tolerance test (GTT). Usually information of equivalent value can be obtained by going off all forms of sugar, refined carbohydrates, starches and stimulants for at least 15 days. This is less expensive and less stressful and is really more definitive than the GTT. If changing what you eat improves the way you feel then why take the GTT?

Look at it another way. If you take the GTT and it shows you have low blood sugar, what did it improve, you will still need to go on a program to improve the way you feel. If you are told the GTT looks like you don't have low blood sugar but you still have the symptoms what do you suggest doing? Our findings are that still the only thing to do is go on a LBS program to see if the symptoms decrease or disappear, and if they do, keep following the program and enjoy your life.

I am sorry to say that I had the test three times. It didn't give me any new information or help me control my blood sugar any better. Even though I knew I had LBS because of how I improved when I followed a LBS program, I still went like a little puppy dog to a doctor and asked for the GTT so the condition could be verified and I could get treatment and care. I got the verification but there wasn't anything a doctor could do about the treatment or care so it was a waste of time, effort, money and hope. To control LBS everyday of your life requires the collection and application of the correct information. The only person on the planet earth who can do these two things is the LBS sufferer. If you haven't learned this yet, learn it now and get on with your life and its fulfillment.

TALK WITH OTHER LOW BLOOD SUGAR SUFFERERS— FOR SUPPORT

You have heard the saying "misery likes company." Well, in the case of a LBS person it's not so much you are looking for company as for comfort and help to make the misery go away. If there is one person in this world who will know how you feel the chances are that it is another LBS person. Maybe for the first time you will have that rare comfort in knowing that you are not the only person who feels the way you do.

We are not saying for one moment that this will lessen your problems, but it will at least give you the opportunity to see your own suffering in another dimension through the other person. Before you know it, you will sound like a couple of old soldiers telling war stories about LBS and its ramifications. Just think if we could have a national convention once a year for LBS people, what a blast that would be if we all went off the program together for the week of the convention. Of course if you haven't started the Krimmel Program yet, you may not be able to see the humor of the thought.

The most special role other LBS people can play is being available when support is needed—and it may be. Don't hesitate to ask them for help. Of course if you can get 4 or 5 LBS people together on a biweekly or monthly basis you will find yourselves swapping recipes, hints and little intricacies which may have taken you years to discover on your own. There is a natural bond that can exist between LBS sufferers that would generally not be there without that common ground. You are very valuable to other LBS victims and they are very valuable to you.

There are cases where whole families have teamed up together and become very supportive to all LBS members of the families.

Some of the most supportive things that can be done with other LBS people are:

Lend and borrow books and articles on LBS.

Trade recipes.

Exchange ideas, hints and personal discoveries on how to deal and live with LBS satisfactorily.

Be available to each other for those times when a supportive person is needed, for there are those times.

The chances of you boring another LBS person while talking about your common condition is fairly slight. You will find, however, that talking about LBS can become a crashing bore to non-LBS people— so please be careful to treat the subject gently with non-LBS individuals, you can avoid a lot of stressful feedback this way.

GETTING OTHERS OFF JUNK FOOD

By "junk foods" we usually mean those that contain sugar and white flour and/or have very little food value. The major reasons these foods enjoy such popularity is that they are made to appeal to the eye and the taste buds. The popularity has nothing to do with their nutritional value or keeping our bodies healthy.

Sugar has no nutritional value, it has no vitamins or minerals only empty calories. The beets, cane or corn that the sugar is made from have lots of vitamins and minerals, but by the time these foods are refined to the sugar state all nutrients have been lost.

In order for the body to metabolize and utilize food there must be certain vitamins and minerals present. Foods in their natural state have all the elements in them that are needed for the body to metabolize and utilize them. Sugar, on the other hand, has no vitamins and minerals in it, therefore in order for it to be metabolized it must use vitamins and minerals from other food previously eaten. This can lead to a deficiency of certain vitamins and minerals such as vitamin B complex.

White flour is made from refining wheat grain, which is high in vitamins and minerals. During the refining process most of the vitamins and minerals are destroyed and/or removed when the germ of the wheat is removed. By Federal law, *some* of the nutrients which were lost must be replaced. This refined white flour is then sold as enriched flour.

White flour is converted to glucose very quickly in the body and increases the blood glucose too rapidly—this is a special problem to LBS victims.

Since white flour and sugar are usually used together you can see why blood glucose will rise very quickly and cause problems for the hypoglycemic.

Some people can stop using all types of sugar "cold turkey," on the other hand, don't get upset if someone has to go off slowly. The objective is to eventually stop using all types of sugar and white flour within a reasonable period of time.

There are various ways to rid the kitchen of sugar and white flour. You can use what you have and not buy any more or you can just throw it all out.

In order to keep junk food (foods containing sugar and white flour) out of your kitchen, be sure you're not hungry when you do your food shopping. Hunger decreases your self discipline and traps you by making all the unnecessary foods look very appealing.

If one decides to go off sugar slowly, then decrease the amount of sugar you use, such as on cereal by ¼ of a teaspoon every few days. In any recipe that calls for sugar, cut it by ¼ the amount each time you make it, until you reach the least amount you can use and still enjoy the item. When decreasing sugar we increase any flavorings, especially vanilla, cinnamon, nutmeg, ginger, etc. to compensate.

We use concentrated (frozen) fruit juice in place of regular sugar when we bake because it has nutritional value and is possibly metabolized slower than sugar. In a recipe that calls for 1 cup of sugar we use about ⅓ cup of thawed juice as a sweetner. Stay away from store-bought sweets because you can't control the amount of sugar in them. The lack of control can put you out of control.

When using flour, gradually change from white flour to 100% whole wheat flour (stone ground rather than steel-roller ground, which is thought to destroy some nutrients because of the heat that the rolling process produces). Substitute a cup, less 1 tablespoon, of 100% whole wheat flour for each cup of white flour that is called for. Each time you make the recipe, increase the amount of whole wheat flour while decreasing the amount of white flour until you use all whole wheat flour. You can use 100% whole wheat pastry flour for a lighter product. Oat, rye and soy flours are even better than wheat flour for a hypoglycemic. I use a combination of 100% whole wheat, rye, oat and soy flours. You can add 1 tablespoon of soy flour in the bottom of each cup of wheat or oat flour that you use. You usually cannot use oat flour alone to replace white flour. See our LBS cookbook for additional ideas.

If you love ice cream, here is a good substitute. Blend 1 cup of milk, 1 cup frozen strawberries (without sugar), 1 tsp. vanilla and ¼ cup non-instant dry powdered milk. Add 2 ice cubes and blend until cold and drink. Or you can leave out the ice cubes and freeze it in the freezer, stir it a couple of times before it is completely frozen for a delicious spooning dessert. You can also do this with peaches.

Coke is a big hang-up with us. But I think it is the carbonation that we like, so we now drink fruit juices diluted with naturally carbonated water (Poland water, Pierre water). At the health food store you can usually find several fruit jucies that don't have any sugar added. It is best to stay away from grape and apple juice, since they are too high in natural sugar even when diluted. Also try adding lime or lemon juice to the carbonated water.

When you want something sweet, try a small amount of fresh fruit. Nuts and carrot sticks are good when you just want something to chew on in place of pretzels, potato chips and popcorn. Nuts must be eaten in small quantities because of high fat content.

Sometimes when you crave sweets it's just that you are bored or frustrated. Rather than eating, go for a walk, bike ride or do some other type of exercise. Too often, food is used for a situation pacifier. You should look at food as a valuable tool for living rather than living to eat.

DAILY REVIEWS AND CHECK LISTS

The purpose of this section is to enable you to improve upon your gamesmanship (the art of winning games without actually cheating) in dealing with low blood sugar on a day to day basis. Even though correcting and maintaining your blood sugar is not a game and should be taken very seriously, there are times when you will find it helpful to have a sense of competition with your own body chemistry. This will involve mostly the tug-of-war between what you want—no matter what the reason—and what is required for maintaining a healthy body chemistry.

A cruel reality is that sometimes your desires stem from, and are controlled by, your body chemistry. A harsh and conspicuous example is a drug addict and/or alcoholic whose body chemistry is dictating what his desires are. The opportunity for him to use his free will has been severely degenerated.

No matter what degree of faulty body chemistry you may have, the chances are that for a long time you have been surrendering to various unhealthy foods and stimulants. Too often people have said to us: "I can't give up drinking coffee, smoking or eating sugar." They have surrendered their own free will. That is why it is often difficult to help those with a faulty body chemistry.

We hope the following schedule and check lists will help you to imporve your gamesmanship in dealing with your LBS.

Sample Schedule

This sample schedule is to act as a guide in helping you lay out your day's schedule. LBS victims must strive to have well-planned, orderly lives with as little distress as possible.

Because of your own particular lifestyle you will need to change our times for your specific times. The important thing is to keep the time intervals and theme as close to ours as possible. We scheduled exercise in the evening but you can do it anytime you feel good and is convenient to you. Write your own schedule on a 3 × 5 card and carry it with you as a reminder.

> 6:00—snack, meditate and exercise in bed
> 6:15—breakfast
> 6:30—shower and dress
> 8:00—snack
> 9:45—snack
> 11:30—lunch
> 12:15—relax for 15 minutes (walk, nap, read, meditate)
> 2:00—snack
> 4:15—snack
> 6:30—dinner
> 8:00—exercise (walk, swimming, calisthenics etc.)
> 11:00—snack and bed

Salt and pepper your day with humor, fun and laughter as often as possible. It is the type of spice that can make life extra nice.

Check List for Daily Review

This check list is to complement your daily schedule. A large part of your success in achieving and maintaining a stable blood sugar is doing the correct things at the correct times. The check list is a means of reviewing your discipline and success in following your daily schedule.

If you can think of any additional support systems we strongly encourage you to use them.

At end of the day, place a check by requirement completed.

REQUIREMENTS	DATE					
Snack before arising						
Exercise before arising						
Out of bed on time						
Breakfast						
on time						
proper food						
proper amount						
Snack						
on time						
proper food						
proper amount						
Snack						
on time						
proper food						
proper amount						
Lunch						
on time						
proper food						
proper amount						
Relaxation						
Midafternoon snack						
on time						
proper food						
proper amount						
Late afternoon snack						
on time						
proper food						
proper amount						
Dinner						
on time						
proper food						
proper amount						
Exercise						
Snack before bed						
on time						
proper food						
proper amount						
Bed on time						

Check List of Don'ts

At this point we are at a list overkill, but we feel we must remind you again and again and again of the things you dare not do if you want to achieve a balanced body chemistry.

Your goal is to develop a lifestyle that doesn't include the items listed below. We realize you may not be able to completely stop all of them immediately. However, you must make every effort to wean yourself off them as soon as possible. If nothing else works, think tough and get angry to regain your free will over your body's chemistry.

Place a check after each item you had. Our suggestion is to do this on a daily basis for the first 2 months and then once a week until you feel you have control of your lifestyle and body chemisry. Your goal is to have no checks and a super balanced body chemistry—this cannot be reached by taking in the various items listed below.

DON'TS DATE						
Additives						
artificial sweetners						
MSG						
sulfites						
Alcohol						
beer						
wine						
liquor						
some patent medicine						
cough syrup						
Caffeine						
coffee						
colas						
cocoa						
chocolate						
tea						
some patent medicine						
APCs						
Sugars—all types						
cake						
candy						
chewing gum						
cookies						
donuts						
danish						
ice cream						
pies						
soft drinks						
Tobacco						
cigarettes						
cigars						
chewing						
pipe						
snuff						
White flour products						
pasta						
bread						

Progress Summary—Symptoms Review

We have found that periodic reviews serve a definite benefit. Once your blood sugar begins to stabilize, there is a strong tendency not to remember where you were and how much you were suffering.

The symptoms list is set up so you can do periodic reviews to see what progress has occurred while following the Krimmel Program. The NOW and 15 days columns have been included so you can have visual continuity of your progress. You may want to transfer your NOW and 15 days information from chapter 3 to this page.

The columns to the right of the symptom list are for reviews after you have been on the program for the given periods of time. Check the appropriate letters:

A = Always
F = Frequently—once or more a week
O = Occasionally—once or more a month
N = Never

NOW A F O N	SYMPTOMS, EVALUATION	15 DAYS A F O N	1 MO. A F O N	2 MO. A F O N	3 MO. A F O N	6 MO. A F O N
	Tiredness					
	Headaches					
	Drowsiness					
	Concentration problems					
	Irritability					
	Sleeping difficulties					
	Dizziness					
	Anxiety					
	Forgetfulness					
	Visual disturbances					
	Depression					
	Fainting/Blackouts					
	Cold hands and/or feet					
	Nervousness					
	Exhaustion					
	Shortness of breath					
	Temper outbursts					
	Sensitivity to light					
	Sensitivity to noise					
	Allergies					
	Muscle pains					
	Phobias (fears)					
	Crying spells					
	Antisocial behavior					

NOW	SYMPTOMS, EVALUATION	15 DAYS	1 MO.	2 MO.	3 MO.	6 MO.
A F O N		A F O N	A F O N	A F O N	A F O N	A F O N
	Asocial behavior					
	Unsocial behavior					
	Suicidal thoughts and tendencies					
	Staggering					
	Craving for sweets					
	Unnecessary and excessive worrying					
	Mood swings (Dr. Jekyll & Mr. Hyde)					
	Nightmares					
	Digestive problems					
	Aching eye sockets					
	Lack of sex drive					
	Impotence					
	Indecisiveness					
	Heart palpitations					
	Internal trembling					
	Mental confusion					
	Undue sweating					
	Bad breath					
	Negative thoughts and attitudes					
	Feeling of going mad, insane					
	Obesity					
	Restlessness					
	Back ache and muscle pain					
	Sneezing					
	Waking up tired and exhausted					
	Arms and legs or body hurt when first rising in a.m.					
	Feel best after 7 p.m.					
	Gasping for breath					
	Sighing and yawning					
	Convulsions with no known cause					
	Premenstrual tension					
	"Motor Mouth" (constant talking)					
	Hand tremors					
	Accident prone					

Fifty-eight symptoms are listed above. Count your responses to each letter and record the number for each below. This will afford you an easy visual aid to see your progress over the indicated periods of time.

NOW	15 DAYS	1 MO.	2 MO.	3 MO.	6 MO.
A	A	A	A	A	A
F	F	F	F	F	F
O	O	O	O	O	O
N	N	N	N	N	N

Chapter 6

FINE TUNING TECHNIQUES FOR MAINTAINING YOUR BLOOD SUGAR

The overall purpose of this chapter is to help you achieve the additional advantages that are so vitally needed when trying to master the art of one-ups-manship in dealing with the problems of being victimized by low blood sugar. We have found from personal experience, as well as when working with others, that most often the little additional refinements can prove to make a very, very big difference. Too often we have met low blood sugar sufferers who were familiar with the general concept of LBS and were only able to make limited progress. When they adopted these refinements they were able to see significant additional improvement. We wish the same for you.

Don't ride your LBS bicycle with half inflated tires, fill them up and enjoy the easier ride.

THE OFFENSIVE POSITION RATHER THAN THE DEFENSIVE POSITION

One of the harshest aspects of low blood sugar is that it creates stress and is aggravated by stress. Because of this it is highly advisable that you make every imaginable effort to develop a lifestyle which is orderly, well planned and happy—stress free.

We hope our following suggestions will help decrease the stress in your life and help you with maintaining an offensive rather than a defensive lifestyle against the pitfalls of LBS.

Preparation of Convenient Food Parcels

It is very important to prepare convenient food parcels so you can enjoy the offensive position at snack time and/or when traveling. If a hypoglycemic has to wait for or prepare the food when needed, he will fall into a deeper slump and not want, or not be able, to prepare it at all.

Examples of Convenient Food Parcels

Be sure snacks are available in case you need to go out unexpectedly, you can just remove them from the refrigerator and put them into an insulated container without any additional preparation. This type of food is also good for the whole family when traveling so you can avoid fast-food items. This will not only save your health but time and money. Try the following:

- Cheese cut into bite size pieces and placed in small tight plastic containers in refrigerator.
- A good supply of hard boiled eggs—a few shelled and placed in a tight container in refrigerator.
- Plain yogurt in 1 serving (½ to ¾ cup) containers.
- An apple cut into eights placed in tight container in refrigerataor, cut only 1 day's supply.
- Whole grain crackers with peanut butter—wrapped tightly and put in refrigerator.
- Handful-size packets of nuts.
- Single-serving containers of cottage cheese.
- Single-serving containers of fresh fruit cup.
- An orange or tangerine peeled and sectioned in a tight container in the refrigerator.
- Single-serving containers of vegetable juice, V-8 juice or tomato juice.
- Fresh fruits and vegetables washed and stored in the refrigerator in 1 serving containers.

Convenient Equipment for Storing and Carrying Food

- "6-pack" insulated container for carrying snacks.
- Thermos bottles—quart and pint size for soups, vegetable juices and water.
- Styrofoam cooler—picnic size for traveling.
- 1 large and 2 medium-size plastic ice packs, the type you freeze in freezer.
- Plastic spoons, knives and forks.
- Snack-size tight plastic containers.
- Plastic refrigerator storage containers of various shapes and sizes.
- Yogurt maker, family size or two, 1 quart size—less expensive to make yogurt than to buy it.
- Insulated attache case to carry snacks to work.
- Small refrigerator for the office to keep snacks and lunch in.
- Alarm wrist watch to remind you when to eat.

PUTTING ON THE BANDAID BEFORE YOU CUT YOURSELF

This means eating before you feel your blood sugar beginning to dip. You don't want to wait to eat until you begin feeling your sugar level dropping. You should strive to learn your body's timing mechanisms (intervals) and symptoms, then eat at the best time to keep your blood sugar on an even level. Don't be a victim of your blood sugar's peaks and valleys when you can "get the drop on it" by eating properly and on time.

Think of the dipping of your blood sugar as the equivalent of cutting yourself and eating as the equivalent of a bandaid you would put on the cut. Of course usually the bandaid is put on after you cut yourself but we are saying to put on the bandaid (eating) to prevent being cut (blood sugar dipping).

LIVE OFF FOOD, NOT YOUR GLANDS

In order to understand the full significance of this concept we recommend you get an anatomy and physiology book from your library and learn how your body works. Most people, unfortunately, have been taught more about world geography than their body's geography (anatomy and physiology).

Here is what we mean by living off food not your glands. If your brain needs blood sugar (energy) and you do not eat to supply this blood sugar, then eventually the brain sends a message to the adrenal glands to release adrenalin. The adrenalin goes to the liver, which then releases glycogen and converts it to glucose, which is released into the blood stream and carried to the brain. The brain receives its blood sugar, but not from food—from the supply stored in the liver which should be used mostly for emergencies. If you frequently do not eat at proper intervals, then your glands end up working overtime to supply your body with its needs. But if you do eat the correct food at proper intervals your body's needs are met by the nutirents from the foods themselves and your glands do not get exhausted and your stored supply of blood sugar is not depleted.

In our opinion when the brain needs glucose (blood sugar = energy) it becomes easily irritated and the slightest annoyance leads to tremendous mood swings—usually losing one's temper or having an argument for no valid reason. This flare up causes the adrenal glands to release adrenalin, which stimulates the liver, which releases glucose to the brain. The brain receives its glucose (energy) and becomes calm. This whole process transacts in a matter of moments. The glands have supplied the energy rather than the food. It is very surprising to have someone extremely angry or upset at one moment and a few moments later act as if nothing had occurred or is apologetic. The person who is yelled at finds it very difficult to understand the sudden and extreme mood swings. This would not be likely to occur if the proper food had been eaten at the correct times.

Another example of this phenomenon is that the glands can be stimulated by nicotine and caffeine. The brain may already have enough energy, but when you dump a stimulant into your body it hits the adrenal glands and stimulates the liver to release stored blood sugar. The next thing you know, your body is lit up like a pin-ball machine.

With caffeine and nicotine stimulating the release of extra sugar into your system, you probably have too much insulin being released which burns up the sugar too fast and then you want more coffee, another cigarette or sweets to raise the sugar to its proper level. Just imagine the peaks and valleys your blood sugar is being forced into by the use of these stimulants. It's a vicious cycle and a merry-go-round out of control.

No wonder we have so many social problems, with people walking around with their bodies' mechanisms having to function in this fashion. What with all these blood sugars being shot up and down all day long and the mood swings that go with it. A world of pin-ball machines banging against one another. Tilt!

Generally speaking, energy from glandular stimulation results in a jerky, up and down, nervous energy, while eating the correct food results in constant, even and non-nervous energy. Which do you think is the more favorable?

Thinking of it in another way, imagine and visualize a fire being maintained with charcoal bricquets in contrast to one being kept ablaze with paper. The bricquets give a constant, even and dependable source of heat (energy) while the paper gives a sudden flashy burst of flame and heat and then dwindles into a very low flame giving off little heat (energy).

BUILDING BRIDGES

The concept of building bridges pertains to trying to sustain an even supply of blood sugar to your body's systems. People with normal blood sugar levels have slight peaks and valleys. Low blood sugar sufferers have extreme peaks and valleys. Thus comes the concept of building bridges in order to avoid the severe fluctutaions and sustain an even supply of blood sugar. You must make sure you build your bridges by eating your meals and snacks at timely intervals throughout the day. This concept is very much akin to "putting on the bandaid before you cut yourself."

PLANNING AHEAD

One of the most common characteristics we have found among LBS sufferers is that they tend to be nocturnal creatures. In fact the hours between 7 p.m. and bedtime seem to be "magic time" for many. During this time they tend to feel conspicuously better than at any other time of the day. For this reason we suggest you consider using part of this time to plan and prepare for the next day—especially the morning which for many LBS sufferers is the most stressful.

Some suggestions:

- Prepare food packets for the next day's snacks.
- Lay out your clothes for the next day.
- Plan and list your next day's activities and duties, especially morning events.
- This is an ideal time for discussion with family members about various plans and decisions that must be made.
- If you are going on a trip, do the packing and car loading (unless you live in the city!).

VITAL SNACKS

Before Going to Bed

In order to sustain your energy supply during your sleeping hours—you must eat a snack immediately before retiring. We have found plain yogurt to be an excellent bedtime snack. There will be times when you will want to forget or supress the idea of eating this snack—don't do it. This is one of the most important things you can do to help yourself get a good night's sleep. Also excellent for avoiding nightmares.

During the Night

Many low blood sugar sufferers wake up during the night and have difficulty getting back to sleep. If you have this problem, try eating 5 spoonfuls of plain yogurt when you wake up. You must eat them very slowly, put a spoonful in your mouth and let it mix thoroughly with your saliva before swallowing it (savor the yogurt). Afterwards, lie back down and do your utmost to keep a calm, blank mood and frame of mind. This is often very difficult to do because the mind tends to initiate a lot of thought activity at this time for some reason. If you haven't gone back to sleep in 10–15 minutes repeat the yogurt and frame of mind. If necessary you may try some light reading for a few minutes to tire your eyes. If this doesn't work the first few nights don't give up, we have found it almost 100% effective once the pattern is learned. It is best to have this snack by the bed rather than having to get up and walk to the kitchem, the less activity the better. Do not turn on the TV or radio and do not have a cigarette.

If you find plain yogurt not to your liking, try adding a little sugarfree applesauce and cinnamon to make it more tasty.

Before Arising

It is also best to have this snack by your bed or have someone bring it to you, so you don't need to get out of bed before having the snack. After eating the snack, lie back for 5 minutes to allow the food to become effective.

One should view his blood sugar supply as a bank account. You can't expect to take anything (money = energy) out unless you have put something in. Very often low blood sugar sufferers wake up somewhat depleted of readily available energy. This is why you eat a snack before getting out of bed, to deposit some food that your body can use for energy before breakfast.

Many subtle things occur with this snack and if you closely monitor your reactions to the foods you will discover the delight of some subtle insights into yourself and your body's chemistry. For instance, before I have my snack I'll be lying in bed and want to get up. But I can only think about it until after I eat the snack, at which time I can activate my desire to get up and get moving.

Some LBS sufferers wake up feeling completely exhausted and like they had been beaten with a baseball bat, particularly their arms and legs. For these people it is imperative to eat this snack. They might even consider a larger snack and/or staying in bed a little longer than the 5 minutes. This severe morning feeling should not prevail too long if you follow the Krimmel Program conscientiously.

Some suggested morning snacks are:

Plain yogurt, ½ to ¾ cup
Plain yogurt with sugarfree applesauce
Orange, peeled and sectioned
Tomato or vegetable juice, 4 ounces, drink slowly

We suggest that the bedside snacks be kept under ice in your insulated bag so they will be appetizing.

GETTING UP THE SAME TIME EVERYDAY

Here is a dimension of low blood sugar which shows clearly how fickle the condition can be.

Let me tell you about Harry. He got up every morning except Sunday, at 6:30 a.m. On Sunday the deviation in time served as the cause for a full day of suffering for him. Harry, like many other red blooded Americans, viewed his staying in bed to this later hour, 9 or 10 a.m., as his "reward" for his early rising the rest of the week. As a matter of fact, many doctors recommend it. But back to Harry. Usually by early afternoon he would be getting a severe headache having spent a sluggish and listless morning. By mid-afternoonoon stomach upset and nausea had set in, followed usually by a surrender and retreat to bed. If lucky, in a short time he was sound asleep, maybe to awaken later refreshed or to sleep the night through.

Over the years he tried many remedies; aspirin, hot showers and many others, but to no avail. Week in and week out, year in and year out, Sundays were days of misery for Harry. This problem occurred on any other day that he would sleep later than 6:30 a.m.—such as times when he was on vacation or trips.

After having Harry get up at 6:30 on Sunday mornings and eating breakfast immediately, he found that Sundays were no longer days of misery.

A large part of the solution can be explained by basing it on the assumption that by 9 or 10 a.m. Harry had bankrupted his body's supply of energy. By this time his blood sugar had possibly fallen excessively low. We have found that low blood sugar sufferers tend to fare far better if they get up in the earlier hours of the morning— 5:30 to 7 a.m. This may have something to do with primitive man. When his lifestyle had to follow the natural light of the sun, he got up with the sun and went to bed with the sun.

Scientists have acknowledged that the body has timing devices and rhythms that we should relate to. It is therefore advisable to try to learn your body's rhythms and try to structure your lifestyle and activities accordingly, such as the time you go to bed, get up and eat your meals and snacks. These activities should be carried out everyday at the same time as much as possible.

LABEL READING

It is imperative that LBS sufferers learn to read and understand labels on all food products. The reason for being so emphatic about this is that too often prepared foods contain sugar and other ingredients—flour, starches, preservatives, sulfites, artificial colors and flavors, and monosodium glutamate (Accent), a flavor enhancer—which are added to products and may be detrimental to a hypoglycemic.

Labels provide a great deal of helpful information. Some of the information is required by the Federal Food and Drug Administration (FDA); some is included on the label at the option of the manufacturer or processor.

Certain information must be on all food labels:

The name of the products.

The net contents or net weight. The net weight on canned food includes the liquid in which the product is packed, such as water in canned vegetables and syrup or juice in canned fruit.

The name and place of business of the manufacturer, packer or distributor.

On most foods, the ingredients must be listed on the label. The ingredient present in the largest amount, by weight, must be listed first, followed in descending order of weight by the other ingredients. Any additives used in the product must be listed, but colors and flavors do not have to be listed by name. The list of ingredients may simply say "artificial flavor" or "natural flavor" or "artificial color." If the flavors are artificial, this fact must be stated. Labels on butter, cheese, and ice cream, however, are not required to state the presence of artificial color.

The only foods not required to list all ingredients are so-called standardized foods. The FDA has "standards of identity" for some foods. These standards require that all foods called by a particular name (such as catsup or mayonnaise) contain certain mandatory ingredients. Under the law, the mandatory ingredients in standardized foods need not be listed on the label. Manufacturers may add optional ingredients. If you want more information about standardized foods write the FDA or the manufacturer of the product.

Under FDA regulations, any food to which a nutrient has been added, or any food for which nutritional claims are made, must have the nutritional content listed on the label. In addition, many manufacturers put nutritional information on products when not required to do so.

Nutrition labels tell you how many calories and how much protein, carbohydrate, and fat are in a serving of the product. They also tell the percentage of the U.S. Recommended Daily Allowances (RDA) of protein and seven important vitamins and minerals that each serving of the product contains. Nutrition information can help you shop for more nutritious food and plan more nutritionally balanced meals for your family. So read the labels!

Nutrition information is given on a per serving basis. The label tells the size of a serving (for example: one cup, two ounces, one tablespoon), the number of servings in the container, the number of calories per serving, and the amounts in grams of protein, carbohydrate, and fat per serving.

Protein is listed twice on the label: in grams and as a percentage of the RDA.

Seven vitamins and minerals must be shown, in a specific order. The listing of 12 other vitamins and minerals, and of cholesterol, fatty acid, and sodium content is optional.

The Recommended Daily Allowance (RDA) is the approximate amounts of protein, vitamins, and minerals that an adult should eat every day to keep healthy. Nutritional labels list the RDA by percentages. For example, the label may say that one serving of the food contains 35% of the RDA of vitamin A and 25% of the RDA of iron. The total amount of food an individual eats in a day should supply the Recommended Daily Allowance of all essential nutrients.

Nutrition labels show amounts in grams rather than ounces, because grams are a smaller unit of measurement and many food components are present in very small amounts. Here is a guide to help you relate to them.

1 pound (lb.) = 454 grams (g)
1 ounce (oz.) = 28 grams (g)
1 gram (g) = 1,000 milligrams (mg)
1 milligram (mg) = 1,000 micrograms (mcg)

When beginning to read labels you will be surprised how many products have sugar added in some form. Almost all canned foods (fruits, vegetables, juices, soups, catsup, etc.), lunch meats, hot dogs and many frozen foods have some type of sugar added. You must also be aware of starches and flour being added to many foods you wouldn't suspect.

Following are some of the names of various sugars you will find on ingredient lists:

Barley malt	Galactose	Mannose
Black Strap Molasses	Glucose	Maple syrup
Cane syrup	Glycerin	Molasses
Caramel	Hexitol	Natural sweeteners
Caramel coloring	Honey	Rice syrup
Corn syrup	Lactose	Simple syrup
Corn syrup solids	Levulose	Sorbitol
Dextrin	Licorice	Sorghum
Dextrose	Malt	Sucrose
Disaccharide	Maltose	Syrup
Fructose	Mannitol	Xylitol

If you read labels on so-called "sugar free" products you will most likely find one of the above sugars on the ingredient list. Therefore, the product is not sugar free—just free of sucrose, the most commonly known sugar.

Your label-reading attitude should be extended to include all medications whether prescription or non-prescription. Many medications, especially cold and cough syrups and lozenges have alcohol and/or sugar in them.

Very interesting isn't it.

EATING OUT

Too often a hypoglycemic will overreact to the fact that he has to be extra careful when eating. The classic comment is, "I won't be able to go out to eat anymore." Nothing could be further from the truth, however you will just have to follow some definite guidelines. Since *adjustment is the height of personal intelligence* we have all the faith in the world that you can make the adjustment.

Eating anywhere other than at home (restaurants, friends' homes, picnic, hospital, air and train travel) does require some additional effort on your part. But it doesn't have to be a traumatic event and you shouldn't become a recluse just because you need to be watchful of what you eat. By keeping a few facts in mind you can enjoy eating out no matter what the setting.

Just as when eating at home you must still be aware of the following items to avoid.

- Any food with any type of sugar.
- Any food with white flour.
- Any food with monosodium glutamate (Accent), a flavor enhancer commonly used in Chinese foods. Ask that it not be added.

Some Tips for Eating in Restaurants

Pick your restaurant carefully—one with a varied menu including foods you are permitted. Consider going to a better restaurant even though it is more expensive with the trade off of eating out less often. You gain at least three advantages by doing this. First, chances are the food preparations are more varied, therefore you have a better chance of getting unbreaded, broiled food in contrast to fried, breaded items. Second, they are more likely to cater to your needs and desires on request. And third, the surroundings and service will probably be more pleasant, which will lead to a greater and more lasting psyche satisfaction.

Take your time selecting food. Don't allow yourself to be intimidated by the waiter, friends or anyone else. If you have any questions about the ingredients of a dish, ask. If you say you're not allowed sugar you have a better chance of getting an honest answer than you do if you say you are a hypoglycemic, which is a bit nebulous to most people.

Following are some suggested menu course selections:

Appetizers
Fresh fruit cup
Shrimp cocktail with horseradish or lemon
Tomato juice
V-8 juice
Oysters on the half shell
Steamed cherrystone clams

Soups
Consomme
Vegetable
Most soups have sugar and/or flour added—be careful

Salads (Take your own dressing or ask for vinegar, lemon and oil.)
Antipasta
Tossed
Chef
Tomato and lettuce
Tomato stuffed with cottage cheese

Poultry
  All—baked, broiled or roasted, no gravies, sauces or breading
Meats
  All—baked, broiled or roasted, no gravies, sauces or breading
Fish and Seafood
  All—baked or broiled, no sauces or breading
Eggs
  Quiche
  Omelet
Vegetables (Order without sauces and ask if sugar has been added.)
  Green beans
  Asparagus
  Very, very small potato, baked or boiled
  Spinach
  Zucchini
  Carrot and celery sticks
  Broccoli
Breads
  Preferably none, especially if you have potatoes
  If you must, then try for rye or whole wheat
Desserts
  Fresh fruit cup
  Apple with cheese
  Melon
  Strawberries
  Nuts
Beverage
  Water
  Herb tea—take tea bag with you and ask for hot water
  Seltzer water with lemon

Food Tips for Vacation, Trips and Picnics

When going on vacation, day trips or picnics it is a good idea to carry some food with you. It is convenient, less expensive, and you have the food you like. Having a cooler and freeze packs enable you to carry a variety of foods for an extended period of time. Here are some foods and equipment suggestions that may prove helpful.

Whole grain crackers
Plain yogurt
Applesauce
Hard boiled eggs, shelled
Whole grain bread
Milk
Cheddar cheese
Nuts
Condiments

Peanut butter
Fresh fruit
Carrot and celery sticks
Butter
Dry whole grain cereal
Vegetable or V-8 juice
Pieces of cooked turkey or chicken
Paper plates, cups and napkins
Plastic spoons, knives and forks

6-pack insulated container for carrying food to short events—shopping, Sunday drive, sporting events, boating, etc.

If Invited

If you casually let your friends know that you aren't able to eat sugar, then they will know how to adjust when they invite you to dinner. If they serve vegetables that are on your no-no list, just take a very small portion and go heavy on the permitted foods. Don't make a big ado and say you aren't allowed to eat those vegetables.

If you are asked about vegetables you do not eat, mention such things as potatoes, rice, corn and beans. Most people can adjust their menu planning around your food needs if they are interested. Make copies of your permitted food list to give to friends who indicate an interest.

Don't make eating the center of your life—eat to live, don't live to eat. Make socializing the important event rather than the food and drink. Don't be conspicuous or make an issue about what you do or do not eat. Your friends, relatives and everyone else simply don't want to hear it, so keep it to yourself, it's your condition.

Also be aware of pressure to eat foods you shouldn't. Just say, "no thank you," and don't make any explanation. If you do have to take it just don't eat it. This way you stay in control of the situation.

If you do make an issue of not eating certain foods and later decide to eat some because you want to cheat a little, you'll find you'll be treated in a variety of negative ways. Better to keep your mouth shut—except for eating what you should eat.

Chapter 7

DIET ANALYSIS
AND
FOOD SUPPLEMENTS

This chapter contains some additional ways to improve your body chemistry and well-being. These logistics can be beneficial, whether you are a LBS sufferer or not—something for everyone's well-being.

DIET ANALYSIS

A diet analysis is a thorough review of your eating habits in relation to quantity and quality. The general procedure is that you fill out a questionnaire which includes a diet survey, health factors and physical activities.

You list the amount of the various foods you eat on a daily, weekly or monthly basis. Health factors include such things as history of diseases, medications, smoking and cravings. Physical activities are a survey of the types and extent of activities you participate in.

A diet analysis should inform you if you are eating the proper foods to be getting enough nutrients and calories for your age, sex and activity level. It should tell you what to do and how to improve your eating habits if needed.

FOOD SUPPLEMENTS

Food supplements are nutrients that are added to our regular food intake to make up for the nutrients that are low in our diet or are needed in larger quantities than usual. Generally speaking, supplements are vitamins and minerals taken in the form of pills, powders or liquid and come in natural or synthetic preparations.

What Are Vitamins?

Vitamins are organic substances found in plant and animal tissues and are needed for body maintenance and transforming food into energy.

They are generally classified as being water soluble or fat soluble. The water soluble vitamins are usually measured in milligrams and are not stored in the body, the excess is excreted in the urine. The fat soluble vitamins (A, D, E, K) are measured in "International Units" (IU). These vitamins are stored in the body and therefore you must be more careful than with water soluble vitamins not to take too large an amount which may build-up to a toxic level.

What Are Minerals?

Minerals are inorganic substances that have been formed in the earth by nature (iron, copper, calcium, zinc etc.) and have two general body functions, building and regulating. They are found in your bones, blood, muscle, tissue, teeth and nerve cells. Their regulating of functions include such systems as the heart beat, blood clotting, maintenance of the internal pressure of body fluids, nerve responses and transport of oxygen from the lungs to the tissues.

VITAMIN AND MINERAL DEFICIENCIES—RELATED HEALTH PROBLEMS

Nutrients (fats, proteins, carbohydrates, vitamins and minerals) work together to keep us healthy and fit. But if only one is missing or low it can cause slight to serious problems. The following are some classic examples of health problems resulting from vitamin and/or mineral deficiencies.

In the days of wooden ships and iron men many British sailors would come down with scurvy on long voyages. They would have swollen and bleeding gums, tenderness of their joints and muscles, bruise easily, scales on their skin, weakness and poor healing of wounds. No one knew why this occurred until Dr. James Lind took an interest and discovered that if citrus fruit was carried on these long voyages scurvy did not occur. Thereafter limes were always provided on these trips and British sailors became known as "Limeys."

It was later discovered that it was the vitamin C in the limes that prevented scurvy. Vitamin C also works to enhance the absorption of iron, and poor iron absorption can led to anemia, which could complicate scurvy.

Beriberi is another condition caused by a deficiency of only one vitamin, thiamine (B_1). In infants, beriberi can cause convulsions, respiratory problems and gastrointestinal difficulties. Adults have fatigue, diarrhea, appetite and weight loss, paralysis, wasting of the limbs due to disturbed nerve function, swelling and heart failure. It is found mostly in the Far East because the basic diet consists mainly of polished rice, which does not supply sufficient thiamine. At times it can be found in other countries when a person's need for thiamine increases due to stressful situations such as infections, pregnancy and alcoholism.

At one time, goiter, an enlargement of the thyroid gland, was very prevalent in the U.S. until it was discovered one of the causes was too little natural iodine in the diet. Since seafood and soil along the coast are high in iodine, people living in these areas didn't get goiters caused by iodine deficiency. When iodine was added to salt because of a federal requirement, goiters were practically eliminated from the general population.

A condition caused by a deficiency of the B vitamins is pellagra. Thiamine (B_1), Niacin (B_3), and riboflavin seem to be the ones particularly involved. Its symptoms are diarrhea, loss of appetite and weight, reddened and swollen tongue, weakness, depression and anxiety (sometimes diagnosed as a mental condition). Itch dermatitis on the hands and neck may also occur. It can be cured with a diet high in niacin, thiamine, riboflavin, folic acid and B_{12}.

Rickets is usually considered a childhood disease caused by a deficiency of vitamin D, calcium and/or phosphorous. The bones of children with rickets become soft and deformities result when the bones try to support weight which they are too soft to do. The bones are soft because they do not retain calcium. Thus children with rickets have bowlegs, knock-knees, protruding breast bone and narrowed rib cage. They may also have tetany and decayed teeth. Vitamin D, calcium and phosphorous work together and if one is missing or deficient it may result in rickets. Vitamin D aids in the absorption and use of calcium and phosphorous. Vitamin C helps the bones retain calcium and phosphorous.

To a large extent all of the above health conditions have been arrested in the U.S. However in some quarteres of the world they still prevail. How many other health difficulties have their answers lurking in the shadows of medical research? It is evidenced by much recent research, that the vast majority of personal medical ills are rooted in a deficiency of or the need for more than the usual expected amount of vitamins and minerals.

DO WE NEED VITAMIN AND MINERAL SUPPLEMENTS?

The need for taking vitamin and mineral supplements is a highly debated subject. Let me tell you one of my personal experiences in taking vitamins and minerals even though I had always eaten a well balanced diet and you draw your own conclusion.

Over a period of 8 years I had a gradual deterioration of my finger and toenails to the extent that I was left with only 2 fingernails and 8 toenails. This had been traditionally diagnosed as psoriasis and treated with various ointments and creams to no avail other than watching one nail after another disappear. After having taken supplements for about a year I was very pleasantly surprised to notice that I was regaining my nails. This was an unanticipated benefit of taking the supplements.

Guess what, I was feeling better than I had in years and being human I began to rationalize my own personal value of needing supplements and stopped taking them. A few months later I slowly started to lose my overall feeling of well being and the nails began deteriorating as well. Needless to say, I began taking my supplements again and lo and behold, as sure as there are little green apples and red ones too, me and my nails are smiling again. All along I had been eating a well-balanced diet, but only with supplements did I improve.

Even though the other members of my family were eating the same foods I was, they did not lose any finger or toenails, therefore it is very obvious that I had some very definite nutrient needs quite different from the other family members. It must be remembered that each individual has different nutrient needs because they are different biochemically, due to:

Age	Ability to digest and utilize food
Heredity	Environment—pollutants,
Activities	temperature, etc.
Mental stress	Physical stress—infections,
Nutritional status	operations, injuries, etc.

Most often we hear that if you eat a well-balanced diet you will get all of the vitamins and minerals you need. Eating a well-balanced diet may have been sufficient when most people grew their own food and ate it fresh or dried and used the whole grains for flour and cereals.

Since vitamins and minerals are so plentiful in nature, the more natural (raw) foods you eat the more chance you have of getting an adequate supply of them. However, any minerals that are not present in the soil where the food is being grown will be missing from that food.

Also, many vitamins and minerals decrease or are lost during storage and when heated to high temperatures. It has been established that if you use a "no water method," steaming or stir frying methods, to cook your vegetables you will retain many more of the vitamins and minerals. Since the water left after cooking your vegetables contains some of their vitamins and minerals it can be used in gravies, sauces and soups rather than being poured down the drain.

The more refined (processed) a food is, the more vitamins and minerals that are lost. Flour made from the whole grain of wheat is high in protein, B vitamins, fiber and other vitamins and minerals. But when it is refined into white flour the germ (where the nutrients are) and bran are removed to be sold separately or fed to cattle and pigs. After it is refined it is also bleached, a process which removes more nutrients. Then it is "enriched" by adding some of the removed nutrients. Why not leave the nutrients in the flour and have whole wheat flour—because somebody decided that besides white flour looking better and storing better you could also make more money by selling the wheat germ and bran separately.

The adulteration of much of our food stuff is a result of our universities and Department of Agriculture cooperating with the food industries for a collection of purely economic reasons rather than healthful reasons.

In our opinion you get few really fresh foods (after a fruit or vegetable is picked it loses nutrients each day) or unprocessed food (nutrients lost during processing) and therefore vitamin and mineral supplements are often required to replace those vitamins and minerals lost.

VITAMINS AND MINERALS—SOURCES AND FUNCTIONS

Below are listed all the primary vitamins and minerals along with what they do and the foods they are found in.

VITAMINS

- Vitamin A—necessary for new cell growth and healthy tissues and vision in dim light. Strengthens cell walls, thus providing mucus membranes defense against infections.
    sources—green and yellow vegetables, yellow fruits, liver, milk, eggs and fish liver oil.
- B Vitamins
    Thiamine (B_1)—required for normal digestion, growth, fertility, lactation, normal functioning of nerve tissue and carbohydrate metabolism.
    sources—brewer's yeast, whole grain products, beans and peanuts.
    Riboflavin (B_2)—helps the body obtain energy from carbohydrates and proteins. Necessary for maintenance of healthy skin, hair, nails and vision.
    sources—liver, kidney, yeast, leafy vegetables and whole grain products.
    Niacin (B_3)—vital for the proper functioning of the nervous system and for the healthy condition of all tissue cells. Aids in stabilizing blood sugar and reducing blood cholesterol.
    sources—liver, peas, beans, whole wheat products and green vegetables.
    Pyridoxine (B_6)—necessary for the proper absorption of B_{12}, utilization of protein, proper growth and maintenance of body functions. Also needed for the production of antibodies and red blood cells. Helps release glycogen for energy from the liver and muscles.
    sources—meats and whole grain products
    Cyanocobalmin (B_{12})—necessary for development of red blood cells and the functioning of all cells, particularly in the bone marrow, nervous system and intestines. Involved with protein, fat and carbohydrate metabolism.
    sources—meats and eggs.
    Folic acid—necessary for the manufacturing of red blood cells and the metabolism and utilization of protein.
    sources—leafy green vegetables, liver and navy beans.
    Pantothenic Acid—important for healthy skin and nerves and aids in the release of energy form carbohydrates, fat and proteins.
    sources—organs meats, egg yolks and whole grain cereals.
    Biotin—important for metabolism of fats, carbohydrates and protein.

sources—egg yolk, liver and milk.

Inositol—helps in metabolism of fats and helps prevent the fatty hardening of arteries and protects the liver, kindeys and heart. Vital for hair growth.

sources—whole grains, citurs fruits, brewer's yeast, crude molasses and liver.

Choline—aids in utilization of fats and cholesterol. Essential for the health of the liver and kidneys.

sources—egg yolk, liver, brewer's yeast and wheat germ.

Para-Aminobenzoic Acid (PABA)—aids in the breakdown and utilization of proteins and in the formation of blood cells. Important for healthy skin and acts as a sunscreen.

sources—liver, brewer's yeast, wheat germ and molasses

- Vitamin C—aids in the formation of connective tissue in skin, ligaments and bones and promotes healing of wounds and burns. Necessary in forming red blood cells and preventing hemorrhaging. Helps fight bacterial infections and decreases the effects of some allergy-producing substances.

  sources—citrus fruits, greens, peppers, strawberries and tomatoes (easily destroyed by heat).

- Vitamin D—aids in the absorption of calcium and phosphorus which are necessary for bone formation.

  sources—fish liver oils, egg yolks, milk fortified with vitamin D and sunshine.

- Vitamin E—(Tocopherol)—is an antioxidant and helps to prevent oxygen from destroying other substances. Plays an important part in cellular respiration of muscles, especially the heart and skeletal, aids them in functioning without as much oxygen. Causes dilation of blood vessels which leads to improved blood flow.

  sources—cold pressed vegetable oils, whole grains, greens, whole raw seeds and nuts, and soybeans.

- Vitamin F—(Unsaturated fatty acids)—helps regulate rate of blood coagulation and breaks up cholesterol deposits on arterial walls. Essential for normal glandular activity and healthy skin, mucus membranes and nerves.

  sources—wheat germ, seeds, vegetble oils, such as safflower, soy and corn and cod liver oil.

- Vitamin K—essential for proper blood clotting, normal liver functioning and converting glucose to glycogen.

  sources—K_1 and K_2 are manufactured by the intestinal tract. K_3 is found in kelp, alfalfa, leafy green vegetables, milk, safflower oil and fish liver oils.

- Vitamin P—(Bioflavonoids—citrin, hesperidin, rutin, flavones and flavonals)—necessary for the proper absorption and use of vitamin C, increases the strength of capillaries, helps build protection against infections.

  sources—white segments of citus fruits, grapes, plums, black currants, apricots, buckwheat, cherries, blackberries and rose hips.

MINERALS

- Calcium—aids in building and maintaining bones and teeth, vital for healthy blood and helps regulate the heartbeat. Assists in blood clotting, muscle growth and contractions, and nerve transmission.

  sources—milk and dairy products

- Chromium—required for glucose utilization, may increase the effectiveness of insulin and transport protein in the blood.

  sources—whole grain cereals, brewer's yeast, liver and corn oil.

- Cobalt—part of vitamin B_{12}. Necessary for normal functioning and maintenance of red blood cells and other body cells.

  sources—organ meats, oysters, clams, milk and eggs.

- Copper—involved in the storage and release of iron to form hemoglobin for red blood cells. Involved in protein metabolism and healing. Necessary for proper bone formation and maintenance.

sources—organ meats, whole grain products, almonds, green leafy vegetables and dried legumes.

- Iodine—necessary for the normal functioning of the thyroid gland, helps regulate the body's energy, growth and development.
  sources—seafoods and iodized salt.
- Iron—combines with protein and copper in making hemoglobin, increases resistance to stress and disease, necessary for transporting oxygen and its utilization.
  sources—liver, heart, tongue, lean meat, oysters, egg yolk and green leafy vegetables.
- Magnesium—activates enzymes necessary for metabolism of carbohydrates and protein, aids in absorption and metabolism of other minerals. Aids in bone growth and is essential for nerves and muscles to function properly.
  sources—fresh green vegetables, raw wheat germ, soybeans, figs, corn, apples, seeds and nuts.
- Manganese—activates many enzymes, related to the proper utilization of vitamin B_1, biotin and ascorbic acid. Necessary for normal skeletal development and for nourishment of the brain and nerves.
  sources—whole grain cereals, egg yolks, nuts, peas and beans.
- Molybdenum—part of two enzymes which are necessary for the transport of iron from the liver and the oxidation of fats.
  sources—legumes, and whole grain cereals.
- Phosphorus—aids in most chemical reactions in the body, important for growth, maintenance and repair of cells. Stimulates muscle contractions, including the heart muscle. Needed for normal bone and tooth structure, kidney functioning and transfer of nerve impulses.
  sources—meat, fish, poultry, eggs, whole grain foods, seeds and nuts.
- Potassium—helps regulate body fluid balance and volume, necessary for growth, normal muscle tone and heart action. Aids in converting glucose to glycogen.
  sources—all vegetables, oranges, bananas, prunes, potatoes and whole grains.
- Selenium—works with vitamin E in metabolism, normal growth and fertility.
  sources—bran, germ of grains, broccoli, onions and tomatoes.
- Sodium—works with potassium to regulate body fluid balance, muscle contraction and expansion, and nerve stimulation. Also aids in keeping blood minerals soluble.
  sources—salt, seafood, carrots, beets and most other foods.
- Sulfur—necessary for good skin, hair and nails; works with other substances for carbohydrate metabolism and strong healthy nerves.
  sources—protein foods.
- Zinc—necessary for normal absorption, actions of vitamins and growth and proper development of reproductive organs. Aids in digestion and metabolism, important in wound and burn healing.
  sources—whole grain products, pumpkin seeds, wheat bran and wheat germ.

HINTS FOR BUYING AND TAKING SUPPLEMENTS

Natural versus synthetic vitamins—which should you buy? During the past 50 years essential nutritional elements have been isolated from naturally grown foods and how many more there are that haven't been discovered is anyone's guess. Since natural vitamins are taken directly from their natural source (plant or animal) all of the known and unknown substances such as enzymes, synergists, catalysts, minerals and protein are taken with it. All of the substances remain in their natural ratio, which is the best way for them to work.

A synthetic vitamin usually has the same chemical structure as the natural vitamin but is made artificially and may not contain the additional substances found in the natural vitamin form. It may also contain added sugar, starch and artificial colorings and/or flavorings which may be harmful and are not found in natural vitamins.

We usually suggest buying natural products whenever possible. They usually cost more than the synthetic, which can be a factor. You can do more research on this topic and should make your own conclusion.

Always buy products which are starch and sugar free. They will usually also be free of artificial colorings and flavorings and preservatives.

If you can, find other people who want to buy vitamins and minerals and you may be able to get discounts for buying in large quantities.

Most vitamins and minerals are more effective when taken with your meals, unless otherwise indicated. We find taking a high quality multivitamin and mineral supplement very satisfactory. I have found that taking 200 mcg of glucose tolerance factor (GTF) with breakfast and dinner helps me avoid hunger attacks and dips in blood sugar. GTF is said to be essential for the proper functioning of insulin and necessary for proper carbohydrate metabolism.

Another aspect is that there are some supplements you should not consider taking, a good example is adrenal extract. In other words, don't become a "supplement popper" just for the sake of taking supplements. You must be discriminating when adding something to your body chemistry. This can best be accomplished by reading and reasoning out why you are doing certain things.

Let us leave you with one lasting thought. The taking of supplements is highly personalized. A good nutritionist or a nutrition-oriented doctor can give you some guidance on what to take, but you should be the one to make the final decision predicated on how you feel after taking the suggested supplements for an extended period of time.

There are some supplements which may help protect you from degenerative and other conditions, and will not necessarily change the way you feel. Only through reading about supplements and how you feel can you formulate your final decision about supplements. Books on vitamins and minerals are available at your library, bookstore and health food store.

Chapter 8

PSYCHOLOGICAL ASPECTS

The way we think, function and act in relation to our physical and social environment is largely a result of how well our body chemistry is balanced. Once your blood sugar is stabilized you will find that your physical and social behavior is greatly improved. For example, you will no longer be frequently exhausted, you will be able to work more effectively, you won't feel as if everyone is against you, and you won't be irritable all the time. At long last you will stop being the puppet of cynicism and despair, and smiles and laughter will begin to display a balanced body chemistry and happy spirit.

Even Sigmund Freud, the father of psychotherapy, believed that biochemistry would ultimately be the answer to problems of the human mind.

BODY, MIND AND SPIRIT

Each individual should see himself as an entity composed of three dimensions, the body, the mind and the spirit. Whenever we have worked with LBS sufferers we have shown them that it is necessary to endeavor to heal each of these dimensions. The Krimmel Program is primarily directed toward regenerating one's body. The mind will gradually begin healing and begin to enjoy a greater amount of continuity as the body regenerates and the body's chemistry stabilizes. Usually the only additional counseling that has been necessary in relation to the mind's activity has been a matter of persuading the individual to be patient during the transition that occurs. It takes time for what we call "clouds" that have been looming over an individual's mind to begin to fade away. As these "clouds" are removed a clear and calm thinking begins to be restored. Of course there is also a great amount of joy and excitement being experienced at this time due to the liberation of the mind. Most people we help say they can't ever remember having had such clear thinking processes before.

We are quick to encourage them to take advantage of this luxury of clear thinking. We suggest they do a general review of their overall lifestyle and work toward atonements where necessary. Some of the general areas of review would include: work environment, career plans, domestic setting and relationships, and social life and plans.

It is our observation that often the individual's spirit as well as his spiritual enrichment has been bruised and put aside due to the long battle and battering of LBS suffering. However once the body and mind begin being glued back together it isn't long before the LBS victim, of his own initiative, begins experiencing a perking up of his spirit and in addition begins pursuing a spiritual renewal. This of course may take any number of directions depending on the person's background, whether it be on a one to one basis or the joining of an organization (Church, ethical society or other).

LOOKING FORWARD AND BEHIND

Understanding and following the concepts of this section are not essential to making progress with LBS, but can prove to be helpful and enjoyable. A common phenomenon that occurs with LBS people after they begin making progress is that they forget exactly how they were functioning and feeling before they started the program. We refer to this as the "brain being kind to itself." If your brain were to remember all the stresses put upon it, it would inevitably be crushed by the strain. Mind you, we are not saying you forget everything, but there is a large percentage of incidents and their character which are forgotten. Your mind tends to repress and/or rationalize the quantity and quality of negative incidents.

If you want to have some fun and experience an interesting event to gain some insight about the above statements, consider doing the following. Before starting the Krimmel Program or very early in the program write a pragraph on how you feel and 1 to 3 paragraphs on three of the following subjects which give you the most anguish and/or distraction.

National politics	Your employment
Religion	Taxation
Your domestic setting	Any subject you choose

After writing these paragraphs, put them away in a secure spot, and dismiss what you have written from your mind. On a separate piece of paper list the 3 subject areas you wrote about and keep it with this book. After 90 days of following the Krimmel Program, refer to your list of topics and again write 1 to 3 paragraphs for each of the same subjects plus a paragraph on how you now feel.

After completing the writing, get what you wrote 90 days earlier and compare what you wrote. Have your thoughts stayed the same, gotten negative or become more positive? If you followed the program faithfully for the 90 days it is practically certain you will be happily surprised and feel great about the contrast in improvement you have made. Not only are you feeling better and thinking more clearly about everything and everyone, but you are starting to be at peace with yourself and the world around you.

The exercise of writing down where you were and how you felt when you first started the program in contrast to where you are 90 days later is written proof of the effectiveness of an improved body chemistry. If you do not see any significant improvement and feel no better, chances are you have not followed the program or LBS is not the cause of your problems.

Healing Old Wounds

Another dimension of Looking Forward and Behind is to review your past and think of any instances that were particularly harsh, awkward or embarrassing that may have been caused by you being a victim of LBS. You probably won't be able to get a concise and clear insight to these types of incidents until your blood sugar is stabilized for an extended period of time—3 to 6 months.

The particular types of incidents we are referring to are arguments, misunderstandings, quarrels and just general upheavals with family, friends, coworkers, etc.

Once having redefined these issues and seeing a necessity for an apology or explanation at this late date, we suggest you make every effort to explain to the given individuals the probable root cause— *Low Blood Sugar*. Tell them in simple terms you have found out you have LBS and its effects, and it was the reason you acted the way you did. The one major benefit you will get from this is to remove the distress of the memories of the incidents and heal the wounds.

What's in a Name?

What's the difference what you call what has been wrong with you in the past, you know that changing what you eat improves how you feel; call it anything you want. What is important is that you can feel great—that's the only important thing. And that is what you should be looking forward to, feeling great! Forget about the name and how you used to feel, that's behind you. Feeling great is the goal! Knowing and doing the things that keep you feeling great is the objective. If you know what makes you feel great now and tomorrow and the next day and the next day, then do it—do it—do it and keep on doing it, because that is looking forward! And who cares what it's called.

PAIN AND PLEASURE BARGAIN

In a way, everything can be reduced to a pain or pleasure bargain. Very often you will pursue an event for the pleasure with the knowledge it is going to cause you some pain (inconvenience, discomfort, expense, hardship, etc.) during or after the experience. A perfect example is our writing this book. We knew from the beginning that we would gain pleasure by sharing our thoughts and concepts in this book. However, fortunately we were realistic enough to know that writing a book would require an immense amount of discipline, time and effort which in most aspects can be construed as a form of pain.

How does the pain and pleasure bargain pertain to LBS sufferers specifically? The LBS sufferer must become very discriminating about what activities he allows himself to participate in. He must evaluate the amount of pain (discomfort, expense, inconvenience, etc.) the activity will cause in contrast to the pleasure (rewards) received. And then decide if the bargain is a good deal.

The following are some examples of pain and pleasure situations.

Turn things around in your mind—waiting an hour for an appointment can be painful unless you adopt the attitude that it's not going to aggravate you and you're going to use the hour productively—reading, relaxing, etc. In a sense, you have pulled the plug on the distress of the situation and turned it into a positive event. Once your blood sugar is regulated this becomes much easier to do.

The cost of cheating—often when you eat something or do something you shouldn't just for the immediate pleasure, you may suffer some type of pain later. For example, eating sweets, drinking coffee, or staying in bed too late may lead to some of your symptoms returning. The amount of pain or discomfort may not be severe enough to cause you to regret doing what you did, whatever it was. So it was a pain and pleasure bargain without too much pain and you will consider doing it again. All we ask is—be sure you are the one who stays in control of the bargain. Not your taste buds, or a situation, or another person. You are the one who will pay the price of pain—so you are entitled to the control. It's called, "keeping your free will."

No gain without pain—nationally famous TV minister, Dr. Robert Schuller of the Hour of Power, often speaks of there being no gain in life without pain. LBS sufferers must be aware that in order for them to make the gains of a stable blood sugar they will have pain (frustration, inconvenience, doing without "goodies," reeducating themselves, etc.) in the process. This gain of a stable blood sugar will be at the expense of some pain—however, the pain of LBS symptoms will be removed, the trade off is definitely a good bargain and leads to a life of greater pleasure and productivity.

OFFENSIVE AND DEFENSIVE POSITION

From a psychological standpoint, it is generally agreed that to be on the offensive in a problem-solving event is to enjoy an advantage. This most assuredly holds true when regulating your blood sugar. Consider your circumstances—You have had, and do have, LBS (a body chemistry problem) which has rained havoc on your life and its stability. Not only have you had to contend with the various symptoms of the condition itself but the symptoms have given cause for many other problems—be they domestic, employment, or social. But now you can take up the staff of the offensive and with your new sense of stability choose your own fate for a change.

Now that the rash of symptoms are off your back and not controlling your every move and action you no longer need to feel defensive. You now can control (take the offensive) and plan your immediate and far reaching future with a sense of stability. The way you eat and function lets you be in the offensive position rather than always defending yourself against the wrath of LBS symptoms. You are in control of your blood sugar rather than it controlling you. Try it, you'll like it.

FIND A BIGGER REASON THAN JUST YOURSELF FOR MAKING PROGRESS

Sometimes doing something difficult just for yourself doesn't seem worth the effort. But if doing it is going to also benefit people you love, work with or admire then the effort is well worth it and easier to do. Some people are motivated to help themselves regulate their blood sugar because of their families, while others find their improvement will let them pursue an activity beneficial to others—for example, scout master, Sunday school teacher, volunteer fireman or being a friend to others in need. It is not unrealistic to choose God as being a good motivator so you can fulfill His plan for you—He certainly wants you to live in a shining Temple rather than a tarnished one, a life without symptoms rather than one tarnished with LBS suffering.

It is also very important that you get involved with some projects once your blood sugar is regulated. You must get moving forward again. It's not important how big the project is or even how profitable it may be. It's more important that the project is worthwhile to you, that it's enjoyable, and that you get a healthy tiredness from its pursuit. It may help just to go out and start helping someone. The idea is to get going and to be involved again.

NOTES

Chapter 9

LIFESTYLE

By definition lifestyle means, the way one lives as shown by one's activities, possessions, attitudes, type of home etc.

Invariably when working with LBS victims we have discovered that their lifestyles were in need of repair. They have been neglecting many areas of their life, be it friends, relatives, work associates or others—there is a general deterioration of their capacity to deal with projects and get along with other human beings. And why shouldn't this happen? Why should we expect something different? After all, aren't their brains under attack moment to moment, day in and day out? So all their activities are distorted because of so many faulty, incomplete, confused or wrong messages being sent by the brain.

We would like to give you some suggestions to help you get your lifestyle back in order.

MAKING UP A ROUTINE, SCHEDULE

Because of the too, too many harsh realities associated with LBS and its symptoms, the victim's lifestyle often takes a severe battering. In order to reduce or minimize the battering we suggest you plan your daily routine using the various aids discussed below.

Alarm wrist watch—a very useful piece of equipment if used effectively, for example it can be used to wake you, to remind you to eat snacks on time, and to keep appointments.

Pocket pad—this handy little note pad should be carried with you at all times so you may log in various events, future appointments and other important notations to be remembered. This potentially decreases the stress of having to rely on your memory by taking it out of your mind and putting it on paper for an easy stress free reference.

Reminder calendar—have one calendar at work and another at home by the telephone. They should show the whole month on one page and have at least 1½ inch squares for each day. Write in all appointments, events and activities for the respective days. This way all members of the family know what the others are doing. It relieves you and the others from having to remember and to remind everyone with a net result of less stress. When you are making plans the calendar is there with all activities listed so you know what days are available for other activities.

Daily cheat sheet—this is a slip of paper with one and only one specific purpose—the listing of various duties, appointments and obligations to be performed that day. The items should be listed in a very brief fashion, limited to 2 or 3 words per item. An example of a typical list for one day may be as follows:

School—Susie 8:30
Office—9:00
(leave space for eventualities)
Shoe repair
Lunch appointment—12:15
Pick up glasses
(leave space for eventualities)
Hospital—George 6:00
Dinner—wife 7:30

If the above style is adequate, all well and good, however if you need or desire a more formal layout there is a large selection of pocket-size appointment pads at most stationery stores. The important thing is to get your duties and appointments on paper to free your mind and reduce stress so it doesn't become distress and wasteful of good blood sugar energy.

CLEAN UP YOUR PROBLEMS—DECREASE YOUR STRESS

Having problems and deadlines looming over you for extended periods of time can foster great stress and eventually lead to distressful circumstances. Don't be membered to the group mentioned in the famous quote of Henry David Thoreau (1818–1862) "The mass of men lead lives of quiet desperation." Cast off your bonds and indignation of passive coexistence—whether it be with a person or circumstance. Reach out and make some transitions and allow a new positive mode to prevail. Make changes and improve your life!

One of the best techniques for dealing with problems is to write them down in list fashion. We suggest that you list items, circumstances and relationships that are problems or causing disharmony in your life. The list may range from something very minor such as cleaning out the garage to something as major as domestic problems with your spouse.

Review the list of problems and divide them into those which must be delegated, such as to a lawyer or a family member and those which you can handle yourself. Each of these lists should be divided into lists of what can be solved immediately (within 2 weeks) and those requiring more time.

You now have easy reference to what needs to be done, and when it is, you will have the gratification of drawing a red line through the completed task.

In order to see both sides of your life make another list of all positive circumstances in your life, from learning that LBS was causing your symptoms to the joy of realizing flowers are blooming outside. Not so bad is it?

NOCTURNAL CREATURE—MAGIC TIME

Many people with unbalanced body chemistry are nocturnal creatures. The underlying reason is that they feel best in the evening and night hours. If this is the case with you, use this "magic time" to its greatest advantage. Even to the extent of considering these hours for your most important activities. Of course, only you should be the one to make this decision. Let your magic time improve your time binding.

Here are a couple of examples of individuals who have changed their schedules to complement their most important activities. A computer research specialist, whose responsibilities required the sharpness of his brain, decided to change his working hours from days to evenings so he could apply the best of his energies to the highest priority of his life during his "magic time." Another woman we worked with changed her job from evenings to days so she could use her "magic time" for her social life, which was her valued activity.

HELPFUL CONCEPTS

Because the character of LBS is so nebulous (varied and vague) we have found that little things can often make big differences in your progress toward a stable life. Ponder the following helpful concepts and choose those best related to your needs. You never know when one of them may prove valuable to yourself or a friend.

Work on the Solution, Not the Problem

This concept would be a good standard for everyone to adopt. How you apply your time and solve problems should be the two underlying principles of your daily activities. Effective time usage doesn't require any additional explanation. However, problem solving should be thought out clearly, particularly in the case of LBS sufferers. In order to be an effective problem solver the individual must use his brain effectively. Remember, one of the main side effects of LBS is not being able to use your brain to its highest efficiency. Quite possibly the brain is the first part of the body to be affected when your blood sugar is dipping. The root cause of this situation may lie in the fact that the brain uses only blood sugar for energy and doesn't store it like other parts of the body but requires a constant new supply.

Just ponder this situation for a moment, here you are, subject to LBS, the brain is not able to function adequately when your blood sugar is low, the brain needs energy from blood sugar to define problems and solve them. Therefore, before making any effort to define and solve a problem be certain your brain is receiving enough energy from blood sugar to function efficiently. In other words make sure you have eaten recently or eat immediately.

Now here is a killer, suppose the problem at hand is that you have to remember to eat on time, with the obvious solution being that you have to remember to eat on time. In order for the brain to remember efficiently (on time) the brain needs energy to energize the thought. How can you remember to eat if the brain doesn't have enough energy? Interesting quandry isn't it? Try thinking about it for awhile—but be sure you eat first!!!

LBS sufferers—and other people, too—too often dwell on the problem, rather than concentrating on the solution and persisting until it is reached. Once you have defined the problem, put it aside and think out the various plausible options for a solution. Evaluate them and work on the most plausible one or ones first. In complex situations this requires listing them and numbering them by degree of plausibility, feasibility and value. It is most important that the LBS person remembers to work on the solution only when his blood sugar is at the proper level. Some people find the early part of the day is the least favorable for problem solving and evening the best. If you are having trouble with the solution learn to put the situation aside and return to it another time.

Remember—once you have defined the problem do not keep repeating it. Too often we hear people constantly restating the problem without ever stopping to think out any solutions and trying them. Most often when a person keeps stating his problem he is asking all in earshot to help him.

Nothing Works Better Than the Way It is Organized and Managed

Two of the major difficulties common to LBS sufferers are organizing and controlling the various events in their life. If you want something to work well, you better plan it well and be willing to check it often—even Santa has to check his list twice. Part of planning may be sitting down and writing out a brief, simple plan in outline form. Keep this plan in a convenient location so you can refer to it quickly and easily as needed. This procedure should be followed fatihfully for all important projects and especially for your LBS program. Bear in mind, if you are having difficulty reaching the goal, your plan may not really be organized adequately. *Nothing works better than the way it is organized and managed.*

Does the Difference Make a Difference?

This is a concept which is as thin as air at times and as mighty as the ocean on other occasions. We strongly recommend that you set it to memory and use it as you would a new tool much needed. The sharpness of this .iew tool will increase the more it is used. Try to apply it to all circumstances, but be aware of becoming a bore by talking about it too often.

Let us give you a working analogy to bring the concept into focus.

Imagine a friend telling you he is going to be a couple of minutes late for a planned event. In some cases the lateness doesn't necessarily make that much difference. However, in other cases a couple minutes lateness could result in a catastrophe, so the difference can make a difference. A couple minutes late for a ball game is quite different than being a couple minutes late for a train's departure and subsequently missing it.

Our main reason for informing you of this concept and hoping you will adopt it is to help you master the art of lessening stress in your life. Stress can be a very harsh enemy to LBS sufferers in how it attacks our stability and body chemistry. Stress is normal in everyday life, but if it becomes too great it can lead to distress which should not be part of our everyday life.

Here are additional dimensions to this concept to play with:

Should the difference make a difference?
Will the difference make a difference?
Can the difference make a difference?
Did the difference make a difference?
How does the difference make a difference?

Another area where the difference can make a difference is particular to your eating. Again let me use an example to make the point. There are times after having eaten a meal that I don't feel quite right. Sometimes I even feel a little down instead of up, even though the meal seemed to be of the correct foods. What I have learned to do is eat 4 to 5 spoonfuls of plain yogurt slowly, this additional aid (may be only particular to me) has been priceless in picking me up on many occasions. This surely has been a case of where a little additional insight has made a very big difference. The difference of the yogurt does make a difference.

You Can't Change the World, Only Yourself

For a collection of reasons, LBS sufferers tend to attack the world and people around them for not being what they want them to be. (This is especially true when their blood sugar is low. This can be a very useful signal to you or others (co-pilot) that your sugar is low and you need food.)

But let's suppose you have a personality trait that makes you want to change the world and you also have LBS, our suggestion is just work on changing yourself. Get your blood sugar regulated and stay on the Krimmel Program for an extended period of time and you'll find that the world doesn't look so bad after all—try it you'll like it. I do!

Always Be Going Some Place in Your Life

Always be going some place in your life rather than just living in the past or present. However, be sure you get happiness from the present or you'll never be able to enjoy the future.

Always think toward an objective, whether it be in your domestic, work or leisure environment. Write your objectives down periodically so you can review your progress and up date them. Should any of your objectives seem overwhelming, list the different ways you can divide them into segments that you can tackle one at a time. Smaller parcels are easier to handle than larger ones.

We have found that large problems or objectives overwhelm LBS sufferers—but once reduced to small segments the same problem is not only achievable but appetizing and solving it is gratifying.

Don't let your life become stale, get to know the people you have contact with every day, the mailman, grocer, bus driver, elevator operator, store clerks, etc. You may not feel like talking to these people until you have regulated your blood sugar, but when you have the feeling, don't smother it. You never know what may come out of a new relationship. Feed a human today—we all need time, thought and consideration.

Be Happy with What You Have or You'll Never Enjoy What You Get

The idea of enjoying less more is sometimes a tough axiom to apply. However, if you look at the opposite situation you can see how harmful it is to be possessed by your possessions. Of course, the optimum is to have much available and use little, getting total enjoyment from everything. Isn't that what a 2 or 3 year old does?

How is this important and how does it relate to the LBS sufferer? Low blood sugar individuals should do their best to develop a lifestyle that has as little distress as possible, one of quality, not quantity.

Let's use an example. It is more valuable for you to own a new, dependable, inexpensive car than to possess an old, undependable, luxury car. Because the distress will be less and the less distress allows for a more stable body chemistry, which leads to more emotional room and time for productivity and enjoyment.

Therefore you must make a conscientious effort to regularly review all the things and circumstances in your life and give them a fair evaluation. Those items and circumstances which are in discord must be disposed of, those in harmony are to be cherished and cared for. Subsequently you will create a profile of a lifestyle which allows you, but does not guarantee, to enjoy what you have and to have time and space in your life to contemplate some additional possessions or involvement when desired.

Depollute Yourself of Harsh Intruders

Let's assume there is an ideal body chemistry. What are some of the things we can do to protect it or recapture it? It has been well documented that many of the items used in everyday life can be detrimental to our body's chemistry and well-being. We strongly recommend and beg of you to consider avoiding all or as many of the circumstances and items listed below. Each is an alien force comprised of molecules which are foreign and injurious to your body's chemistry. If it were not so serious it would be hilarious to think about what the modern day human being does to his body with foreign substances.

Most LBS sufferers have allergy type symptoms. These are often brought on and aggravated by various substances listed below.

Perfumes: including fragrances in shampoos, deodorants, lotions, paper products, hair sprays, powders, soaps, laundry softeners, candles, etc.
Smoke: cigarettes, cigars, pipes, incense, industrial, etc.
Household cleaners: oven cleaners, furniture polishes, window cleaners, air deodorizers, toilet bowl deodorizers, etc.
Cooking odors: fish, yeast, charcoal fire starter fluid, etc.
Fumes: diesel and combustible engines, paints, space heaters, etc.

We suggest the avoidance of as many of the above substances as possible. In some cases substitutes can be used. For example, opening windows or lighting a match or an unscented candle to remove odors from a room rather than using an "air freshener" spray. The lighting of a candle or match may seen bizarre, but if you remember basic chemistry, the universe is comprised of three basic substances: solids, liquids and gases—and odors are gases. And what is the number one gas attacker—eater upper—fire, not another gas, such as an air spray.

Read labels when buying soaps, lotions, paper products (tissues, toilet paper) etc. to be sure fragrances haven't been added. A good soap without excessive fragrance is Ivory hand and bath soap.

The best environment is the one with the fewest unnatural intruders. It is amazing that our culture seems to have decided that everything has to be adulterated with either a smell or a color. The chain of events must be broken, whether you are talking about the artificial coloring of oranges or perfumed toilet paper. Talk about a culture going from the absurd to the sublime.

UNDERSTANDING THE ECONOMICS

Beneath the veneer of every organization are the roots of economics. No matter what you call it or what its ultimate purpose may be the economics of the organization must be keenly considered. This holds true to the individual just as it would hold true for the U.S. government and the Vatican City.

Your LBS condition has an economic side also. The LBS sufferer often believes that to change his food habits and lifestyle will result in high expenses, this we do not believe to be the case.

Not More Expensive for Food

Besides being healthier, natural foods will ultimately save you money, too. Once you stop buying the cake, cookies, donuts, potato chips, sodas, fast foods, etc. and buy only fruits, vegetables, grains,

meats and dairy products, your food bill will decrease. Eating unprocessed foods are more filling, stay with you longer and are more
satisfying than the processed packaged and fast food items. Eating a
piece of fruit for a snack is much more satisfying than cake, cookies,
potato chips, etc. Try it, you will like it. And your pocketbook will too.

Fewer Medical Bills

Once a LBS sufferer's body chemistry is stabilized the symptoms
which he commonly had to cope with often lessen significantly, if
not totally disappear. This unto itself leads to a great reduction in his
need for medical assistance. As the weeks and months go by he will
find himself seldom having a need for doctors in contrast to the olden
time situation where he probably was always on the verge of wanting
to see a doctor about his symptoms. And each time he saw a doctor
he was billed whether he improved or not. Of course we are assuming
he was a classic hypoglycemic sufferer—one who staggered through
the medical maze in search of help going from doctor, to doctor, to
doctor.

Income May Become More Stable and Even Increase

We are not saying unequivocally that your income will become more
stable or increase, but you will have a better shot at making money,
because you'll feel better.

As your blood sugar and body chemistry become more balanced,
you begin to feel more stable and function with greater proficiency
which most likely will lead to a greater degree of stability in your
work life and other activities. As you function with greater efficiency
in your work endeavors you should start planning to take advantage
of this new stability you have gained from being on the Krimmel
Program.

Once you have confidence that you are in control of your blood
sugar rather than it controlling you, start thinking about how you
can advance in your work and career. Reach out and pick the fruit of
your efforts and new stability.

> Think as the Seabees.
> Take on the attitude
> of their famous motto;
> *Can Do!*
>
> Decide
> Plan
> Act

Chapter 10

LIVING WITH A LOW BLOOD SUGAR SUFFERER

Much has been written about people with LBS, but little attention has been given to the ones living with them. We who live with them may not suffer as much as the LBS person, but we do suffer because of their problem.

LBS people often keep their "cool" with friends and relatives but with their immediate families they often become intolerant and abusive, verbally and/or physically. What the injured person must remember is that the abuse is not personal. The LBS sufferer is just reacting to his blood sugar being low and not reacting to the individual personally. The insulted or injured individual must learn to put his ego behind him. Nuns and nurses in some settings, because of their duties, are perfect examples of people being able to perform in this fashion. If you allow yourself to react on a personal basis, you have your ego in front of you, you must put it behind you before you can begin really helping a LBS sufferer.

This is very difficult to understand and accept. But to retaliate just makes the situation worse and more difficult for reconciliation. The best thing to do is to give the LBS person some proper food to eat. In a few minutes he will be much more agreeable. Giving food will make a difference.

What must be learned and remembered is that for a person to keep his emotions and temper under control there must be sufficient fuel going to the brain and nervous system continually. This is very difficult for an LBS person. Once this is learned, understood and accepted, then there will be far fewer hurt feelings and more looking for signs of "low fuel," "short fuse" or whatever, so it can be prevented. Each person usually has his own signs, maybe swearing, certain swear words or any special words, certain actions, look in the eyes, lack of concentration, deep breathing, etc. Make up a list for your LBS person and discuss it with him when his sugar is normal.

What can be done to prevent or stop the "attacks?" Have small packets of food available, usually in the refrigerator (see Chp. 6, FINE TUNING TECHNIQUES). Encourage the LBS person to eat some food, hand it to him, and as a last resort, put it in his mouth and walk away. Usually you will only need to put it in his mouth when an attack is in progress. Often you will receive a thanks after his blood sugar returns to normal and he realizes how he had been acting.

You must relate to an LBS sufferer (when his blood sugar is low) as if he were without any sensory equipment. Would you insist on a blind person seeing? One who can't hear—would you yell at him, etc. etc.? When the blood sugar is down, the person most often can't help himself—so why don't you help him—he needs you. What's wrong with needing and being needed?

Mornings are usually a very stressful time for many LBS sufferers and I find it best not to bring up any matters that could be stressful. Try not to plan any activities that are unpleasant for the morning and this leads to a more pleasant life for everyone. The best time for discussions and decision making is usually in the evenings. Try to use this time to its best advantage, but don't take advantage of the LBS person by making him feel guilty about past events.

It sounds as if the family's activities must be controlled by the LBS member, and this may be very much true—in the beginning, until the blood sugar is brought under control. Once the blood sugar has been stabilized for a period of time then the "lows" can be prevented by eating regularly and frequently. In the beginning the LBS person must be given food to eat, then just reminded and hopefully he will in time automatically eat frequently and avoid all lows even in stressful situations.

PILOT-COPILOT RELATIONSHIP

As a spouse of an LBS sufferer I will be eternally thankful for the blessings that we have received in finally finding out Ed has LBS. We have had many additional blessings since that day and one in particular is my having been supplied with enough energy and creativity to work with Ed in understanding and managing his blood sugar. We generally refer to this area of cooperation between us as being the pilot-copilot relationship. There are times when Ed's blood sugar is in a deep dive and only because of this relationship is he spared crashing. For more specifics on pilot-copilot relationship see Chapter 5.

FAMILY MEMBERS MUST LEARN ABOUT
LOW BLOOD SUGAR

As the adage states, *knowledge brings joy.* This is surely true about LBS. The joy of the LBS person and those around him is directly proportionate to the amount of information gained—and applied. We strongly encourage each and every person to make a definite effort to learn the concepts and insights of LBS. The benefits and rewards will be infinite. Reading is the most reliable means to this end. But along with the reading you must observe and learn the LBS person's individual symptoms, signs and characteristics of when his blood sugar is causing problems. Also you must learn what foods are best for him in controlling his blood sugar.

However, let me caution you that no matter how much you read and no matter how much you learn, it will all go for naught unless you apply it patiently and consistently with as much understanding and love as possible. Let your understanding and love pour free!

We suggest the family sit down as a unit and have discussions periodically about the progress being made or not being made. This effort is not for the purpose of making the LBS person feel defensive but to let him know his progress is valuable to the whole group and that they want to be supportive. An ideal way of airing negative comments is to have all comments submitted in writing rather than verbally. It is a good idea to change the chairperson each time. In some cases it may be a good idea to keep a log of the pertinent points made at these meetings.

You will find it valuable to have contact with other LBS people and their families. You will gain insights, ideas and support from these individuals.

FAMILY MEMBERS SHOULD BE WILLING TO CHANGE EATING HABITS

Sayings such as: *Your body is your temple; You are what you eat: Where are you going to live after you wear out your body?*, are often ridiculed and may seem simplistic until we have a specific reason for wanting and needing to relate to them. Once an LBS sufferer begins making progress he will be able to relate to them very easily.

The food ethic of the Krimmel Program is of such a high quality that no one should have any qualms about following it if they are interested in a quality and healthy lifestyle. It is good for the whole family, not just the LBS member.

There are distinct advantages for everyone following this ethic:

Supportive: It is supportive to the LBS member and rids the immediate environment of all the harsh intruders (sugar products, tobacco, caffeine etc.) on the LBS person's health and stability.

Economics: Planning one menu for the family is less expensive than planning two menus. Also, you will not be paying for any junk or fast foods, and your food costs will probably decrease. Cutting out cigarettes and alcohol could save $300 to $2,000 per year.

Reduce risks: Since LBS and diabetes seem to have a tendency to run in families, everyone following the program will decrease his or her chances of getting the conditions or decrease the severity of them. LBS appears at times to be a precursor of diabetes.

Family harmony: Once every family member follows the food ethic there appears to be more harmony and less bickering, although we don't have any related scientific evidence concerning this. It is an interesting phenomenon that in some families there are more than one having LBS. Once the family is on the food ethic don't be surprised if more LBS people come out of the woodwork. Marge Blevin and Geri Binder, the authors of THE LOW BLOOD SUGAR COOKBOOK, indicated that between their two families there were eight people suffering from LBS. This was one of the underlying factors in their having written the book.

Convenience: Preparing one menu for the whole family is more time efficient and convenient than preparing two menus.

Educational: When following this food ethic some individuals will notice a feeling of well being, particularly if they had gotten headaches or other complaints before beginning the food ethic. This will help educate them as to how certain foods can affect them. Also if a few members start getting some positive feelings and insights it may give everyone some enthusiasm for learning more about food and its relationship to their body.

CHARLES' COMMENTS

I've lived with my Dad and Mom all my life and we have had a great time. We've lived in a lot of places and have traveled all over the United States, mostly due to my father having low blood sugar.

My Dad's low blood sugar condition can cause some hardships:

- We can't have junk food for dinner.
- If his sugar is low and you want to go somewhere he says no.
- When he eats sugar he is very touchy and "spaces out" on you when you do one wrong thing.
- You have to take food with you wherever you go.

But now it's great because he doesn't have the problem much anymore. Also I've learned a lot about what I should and shouldn't eat.

QUESTIONS AND ANSWERS

Q. What is hypoglycemia, low blood sugar?

A. Hypoglycemia is the formal name for low blood sugar, a condition where the blood sugar falls below the range the body requires to function normally.

Q. What is the difference between organic and functional hypoglycemia?

A. Organic hypoglycemia is caused by an organic problem such as a tumor of the pancreas, enlarged pancreas, defective liver, pituitary malfunction or diseased adrenal glands. All of these conditions can cause excessive insulin production which leads to LBS. The most common type of hyopglycemia is functional which is caused by an overactive or oversensitized pancreas but with no pancreatic disease or structural problem. Factors related to functional hypoglycemia are: excessive use of sugar, overactive pancreas, adrenal insufficiency, imbalance of other hormone secretion, excessive use of alcohol, tobacco, caffeine and severe emotional shock or trauma.

Q. Is it true that the average American consumes over 100 pounds of sugar a year?

A. Yes. Many people think they don't eat sugar unless they eat sweets (pie, cookies, ice cream, sugar in beverages) but just look on the ingredient list of almost any food in the supermarket and it will usually have some form of sugar in it. About the only items that don't have sugar added are fresh food and plain frozen food.

Q. What is blood sugar?

A. Blood sugar is the simplest form of sugar and it is called glucose. Glucose is the only form of sugar that can be absorbed and used by the cells in the body.

Q. Why do we need glucose?

A. Glucose supplies all of our body's cells with the energy they need to perform their work.

Q. If glucose is sugar why can't I eat regular sugar (table sugar, sucrose) for energy?

A. Regular sugar (table sugar, sucrose) is so refined that it is metabolized and absorbed into the blood stream too rapidly. The blood sugar (glucose) rises suddenly causing too much insulin to be secreted and the blood sugar is utilized too rapidly resulting in your blood sugar falling causing LBS symptoms. You may have an increased energy level for a short time after eating the regular sugar (table sugar, sucrose) but it will not last long. On the other hand, if you ate some complex carbohydrates such as fresh vegetables or grain products, which are metabolized slowly thereby releasing glucose into the blood stream slowly, your energy level would be sustained over a long period of time.

Q.   Is LBS a disease or what?

A.   LBS is not a disease it is a condition. It is the condition of the body's chemistry being out of balance.

Q.   What would be a one sentence statement of the purpose of the Krimmel Program?

A.   The main purpose is to encourage people to refrain from using refined sugars and starches, all stimulants and to get the proper exercise, rest and relaxation, and fun and laughter.
OR
To change the body chemistry of the individual—one which is more suited to the needs of the human body and brain.

Q.   Are there any times when the blood sugar drops low and is still considered normal for a person?

A.   Yes, there are two general times during the day when an individual's sugar is expected to drop to a low point.
1. Sometime between 10:00 and 11:30 a.m.
2. Sometime between 2:00 and 4:30 p.m.
That is why it is a good idea for everyone to have a mid-morning and mid-afternoon snack, to avoid these low points.

Q.   What can I do if I feel hungry all the time after following the Krimmel program for a few months?

A.   First you must be certain you are eating sufficient calories for your size and amount of daily activity. If you are, then we have found that taking a glucose tolerance factor (GTF) helps relieve this problem. GTF is said to be essential for the proper functioning of insulin and necessary for proper carbohydrate metabolism. It is preferable not to use GFT in the first few months of the program.

Q.   If I am a hypoglycemic and need to be a hospital patient how can I be sure to get the correct diet?

A.   Before you enter the hospital talk with your physician about your diet and even give him a copy of allowable foods to be given to the hospital dietitian. Also when you get to the hospital ask for the dietitian to come see you so you can review the food list and qualify your needs. Don't take a passive position because then you will probably be ignored. Remember, LBS is not looked upon as a credible condition by most of the medical camp.

Q.   Is nutrition taught in medical school?

A.   In the vast majority of medical schools nutrition is not taught as a course. There are aspects of nutrition taught as related to specific conditions such as diabetes, high blood pressure, after surgical procedures etc.

Q. Does a hypoglycemic have to have all the symptoms that are listed in the book?

A. No. It is not so important how many symptoms you have but rather how often they occur, how severe they are and how long they last. Everyone usually has a majority of these symptoms sometime in their life but for a very short duration. Our findings are that those who have hypoglycemia usually have approximately 20–40 symptoms ocurring on a regular basis until they are on the proper program and their blood sugar is regulated. However, if you have only a few symptoms and they are persistent you may have LBS.

Q. Is there a symptom that the medical camp gives more credibility to than any other symptom as being caused by LBS?

A. Yes, our findings over the years indicate that those individuals having the least difficulty being diagnosed as hypoglycemics have one symptom in common—passing out, fainting, blacking out or whatever you want to call it. When blacking out cannot be attributed to any other cause and the physician has looked high and low for an answer, very often he will finally order a GTT for the patient. That is the one luxury of passing out—you have a better chance of being diagnosed quicker than those who do not black out or faint.

Q. What is the likelihood of low blood sugar being an underlying cause of many social and personal problems and difficulties in the United States today?

A. Highly probable! But unfortunately there are no absolutely scientific studies to collaborate this opinion. Just think how much less crime, employment difficulties, domestic problems and health costs we would have if our opinion is correct. Talk about cultural lag!!

Q. Is it true that many "mental conditions" are caused by hypoglycemia?

A. Several psychiatric hospitals have given glucose tolerance tests to their patients and have found that a high percentage of them have hypoglycemia, especially those diagnosed as schizophrenic. After these patients were put on the proper hypoglycemic program their symptoms disappeared and their behavior improved. Much research needs to be done in the area of "mental health" and its relationship to body chemistry.

Q. Do the effects of LBS affect your social behavior?

A. Yes.

Q. Why are people who have LBS often overweight?

A. Often people with LBS have a craving for sweets and they over indulge in these refined carbohydrates (low quality foods) which leads to weight gain. Also many of these people are always tired and feel beaten down therefore they do not exercise and work off those extra calories.

Q. Can a person have episodes of LBS without being a hypoglycemic?

A. Yes, at times of severe stress or just before a woman's menstrual period the blood sugar may drop. Also most people have a normally low blood sugar in mid-morning and mid-afternoon. By taking a healthy snack before these times corrects the situation.

Q. Can a person have LBS symptoms but have a normal glucose tolerance test result?

A. Yes. Just because there are certain levels of blood sugar which are considered normal (80–120 mg.) it does not mean that it is normal for everyone. The most important aspect of a GTT is how fast the sugar drops, if it goes below the fasting and how long it remains there.

Q. How many alcoholics are hypoglycemic?

A. There is no research that affixes absolute numbers of alcoholics being hypoglycemics. However, those physicians who relate to LBS and work with alcoholics find an extremely high correlation between the two conditions. Some physicians have come to the conclusion that all alcoholics are hypoglycemics. Our bottom line is that all alcoholics are first and foremost people with body chemistry problems. Once you accept this premise your first question is "Why aren't all alcoholics given a complete body chemistry work up?" If you ever go to an AA meeting, one of your first observations will be that there is an extremely large amount of sweets, coffee and cigarettes being consumed. Some would say these stimulants are substitutes for alcohol. Think about it.

Q. If my doctor tells me I have LBS, what should I do?

A. No matter how you discover that you have LBS, the most valuable thing you can do is build a very large reservoir of reliable information concerning LBS and body chemistry. The most direct and valid means of achieving this is to read, read, read and talk to other LBS individuals. It is very important to consider the medical dimension of LBS but most physicians do not have the time to give you in-depth guidance and insights required for understanding and maintaining your blood sugar.

Q. Why do hypoglycemics have so many nervous system related symptoms?

A. The cells in the retina of the eye and the brain, which is the center of the nervous system, can not store glucose for energy, whereas the rest of the body can also use fats for energy. Therefore when the blood sugar falls the nervous system is the first affected which leads to nervousness, irritability, headaches, etc.

Q. If I have LBS can I use artificial sweetener to replace sugars?

A.   No, artificial sweeteners promote the idea that everything you eat must be sweet. Also it is not known how the pancreas relates to artificial sweeteners, how does the pancreas know it is not sugar.

Q.   Since many people with high blood sugar (diabetes) take insulin, what medications do people take for low blood sugar?

A.   None—To date the only way to control LBS is through the proper diet, exercise, rest and fun & laughter.

Q.   Does Low Blood Sugar have a hereditary factor?

A.   Low blood sugar has not been proven to be hereditary, but at times it does seem to occur in families.

Q.   How old do you have to be before you can get LBS?

A.   There is no special age. Some premature babies are born with LBS because the control of the blood sugar has not yet been properly balanced by their hormones. There are babies who develp hyopglycemia at a few months but this is not common.

Q.   Can stress cause LBS?

A.   Yes, the stress from such things as surgery, trauma or pregnancy can result in LBS but usually ends once the stress is over. Continual stress over an extended period can be a factor leading to one becoming a hypoglycemic.

Q.   Is it true "once a hypoglycemic always a hypoglycemic?"

A.   No. Some individuals may have a period of hypoglycemia after pregnancy, surgery, trauma or prolonged emotional involvement but when the stress is over usually the hypoglycemia disappears. If the hypoglycemia is caused by an organic problem such as a tumor of the pancreas then when the organic problem is corrected so is the hypoglycemia. Functional hypoglycemia usually does not go away but can be controlled by diet, exercise, rest, fun and relaxation.

Q.   Are table sugar and blood sugar the same?

A.   No. Table sugar (sucrose) is a combination of glucose and fructose, blood sugar is just glucose.

Q.   What may be some contributing factors to LBS?

A.   Excessive use of refined foods, alcohol, caffeine and tobacco, also hormonal imbalance and adrenal insufficiency, and emotional stress.

Q.   What is high blood sugar called?

A.   Diabetes, Diabetes mellitus, Hypoinsulinism and Hyperglycemia.

Q.   What is low blood sugar called?

A.   Hypoglycemia, Hyperinsulinism.

Q.   Can LBS people use honey?

A.   No, since honey is sugar. However, some LBS people seem to be able to tolerate a very small amount of honey in cooked foods.

Q.   What are the most important things I can do if I have LBS?

A. 1. Consult a physician.
   2. Eat the proper foods, exercise and get proper rest.
   3. Read as much as you can find on LBS.
   4. Locate other LBS people and talk with them.

Q. What does metabolize mean?

A. It means how the body assimilates, absorbs, utilizes and burns up the food (nutrients) we take into our body.

Q. Why is it important for family members of a hypoglycemic to understand hypoglycemia?

A. It is usually helpful for all of us to have support when we are trying to succeed in something. Hypoglycemics usually need and appreciate support, and in order for family members to give this support they must understand hypoglycemia. Since the hypoglycemic must not eat certain foods and does need to eat several times a day, the family members may need to remind him when to eat and encourage him to eat the proper type of foods. We usually encourage the whole family to follow the food ethic since it can only do good for everyone. Only through understanding can we help each other.

Q. If I have LBS symptoms but my doctor says my GTT doesn't indicate LBS, what should I do?

A. If there has been no medical reasons found for your symptoms after a thorough medical and body chemistry work up, then follow the Krimmel Program for at least 90 days and see if there is any reduction in your symptoms. If you feel significantly improved then continue on the program and read all you can about body chemistry. Also try to find a physician who is nutritionally oriented.

Q. Is it possible for a person to have both high blood sugar and low blood sugar?

A. Yes. In some individuals the pancreas may be underactive after eating, permitting the blood sugar to rise to a high level, and then the pancreas may become overactive a couple of hours later secreting too much insulin and causing the blood sugar to fall too low. This is one of the reasons if you have a GTT it is important to have a 6 hr. GTT rather than only a three hour GTT. If this type of person had only a 3 hr. GTT only the diabetes (high BS) would show up because the test would be discontinued before the hypoglycemia (low BS) showed up.

Q. What is a normal blood sugar?

A. A normal blood sugar is the level of blood sugar that enables an individual to function without any side effects of high blood sugar or low blood sugar. We must bear in mind that each of us is an individual entity unto ourselves in relation to our body chemistry, what is normal for one individual may not be normal and compatible for another. It's been said, "There is no number,

no point, no range of blood sugar which constitutes hypoglycemia." However, most physicians consider 80 mg. to 120 mg.
as normal blood sugar.

Q. How much alcohol can a LBS person drink?

A. It is best not to drink alcohol at all since it is a fast acting carbohydrate. Many hypoglycemics have liver involvement and
since alcohol is detoxified by the liver this causes additional
stress to the liver. Also alcohol may reduce the liver's output of
glucose. Alcohol definitely interferes with your mental, physical
and social well being and should be totally avoided by all people
and most particularly people with body chemistry problems.
Alcoholic drinks include ale, beer, wine, whiskey, rye, cordials,
rum, etc.

Q. Is hypoglycemia a rare condition?

A. No. Perhaps it was to the caveman but not to modern man.
Since the advent of refined foods, stemming from the industrial
revolution, all degenerative conditions have substantially increased percentage wise. Classic examples of degenerative conditions are heart disease, diabetes, hypoglycemia, arthritis, etc.

Q. If hypoglycemia is not rare why is it so difficult at times to get
it diagnosed?

A. Hypoglycemia's symptoms are also symptoms of many other
conditions. People are usually treated for these conditions first
and if they do not respond to treatment then they may be tested
for hypoglycemia. However hypoglycemia does not enjoy much
credibility in the orthodox medical camp. Some doctors will not
even test for it and even when tested for it by a GTT, the results
may be misinterpreted.

Q. Is the Krimmel Program suitable for all ages?

A. Yes, it is suitable for all ages but must be relative to the age of
the individual. You wouldn't give nuts or seeds to a one year
old, however you should be giving him a diet without refined
carbohydrates and seeing that he gets the proper rest and exercise (play). And don't forget fun and laughter.

Q. Why does the low blood sugar individual have to be careful of
how much fruit juice he drinks and how fast he drinks it?

A. Fruit juices are *very high* in *natural sugars* with grape juice being
the highest. Drinking grape juice is almost like eating sugar
straight and should never be taken by a LBS person. Orange
juice and grapefruit juice may be used in small quantities, ½ cup,
at a time. Some authorities on LBS suggest you should dilute
juice with ½ water. You should sip juice rather than drinking it
right down, it could possibly stimulate the pancreas to release
too much insulin which would use the glucose too quickly
thereby causing your blood sugar to fall rather than maintaining
the blood sugar level with the juice.

Q. Will I get fat on the LBS diet?

A. No, refined carbohydrates and over eating are what usually cause weight gain and these have been eliminated in this diet.

Q. Do low blood sugar and hypoglycemia mean exactly the same thing?

A. Yes, they are used interchangeably. From a technical standpoint hypoglycemia is the name of the condition when the blood sugar is low.

Q. If I have low blood sugar, shoudn't I eat sugar?

A. No, as odd as it may seem, eating sugar results in your blood sugar going low. All sugars are fast acting carbohydrates and fast acting carbohydrates are quickly metabolized and absorbed into the blood stream causing your blood sugar to rise rapidly which may result in too much insulin being released. The insulin causes the sugar to be used too rapidly and the blood sugar falls too low. It is not necessary to eat sugar in order to maintain a normal blood sugar level because blood sugar is derived from carbohydrates and even proteins and fats if necessary.

Q. Wouldn't the Krimmel Program be helpful to just about everyone?

A. Yes, this program would be beneficial to most people, but anyone on a special diet should check with their physician. The Krimmel Program of the proper food, exercise, rest and relaxation, and fun and laughter is just about as fine a lifestyle as you can follow.

Q. Is the Krimmel Program good for losing weight?

A. Yes, because refined carbohydrates, which lead to weight gain, are not included in the diet. Also exercise is very helpful in weight control. However, if you are not overweight, you will not lose weight on this program as long as you eat enough in proportion to your exercise.

Q. Why are there a variety of LBS diets?

A. The original diet by Dr. Seale Harris, the discoverer of LBS, was a high protein, low carbohydrate and moderate fat diet. Most LBS diets are based on his diet, however some LBS authorities have found their patients do better on a high complex carbohydrate, low protein, moderate fat diet. There have been studies that show a high protein, low carbohydrate diet can be detrimental because it over stresses the adrenal glands. Studies also indicate that a high protein diet may contribute to such degenerative conditions as kidney damage, osteoporosis and premature aging.

Q. Are snacks important if I have LBS and eat three good meals a day?

A. Yes. Snacks are one of the most important things you can do to maintain your proper blood sugar level. They build bridges so your blood sugar will not drop between meals. It is vitally important that snacks are high quality food rather than junk food.

Fresh fruit, nuts, hard cheeses and peanut butter (without sugar) are good snack foods. See Chapter 4 for snack suggestions.

Q. Will my symptoms return if I go off of the food ethic?

A. Yes. Of all the hypoglycemics we have talked to and read about their symptoms do return if they deviate from their program. In a sense it is relative to each individual and depends specifically on how severe a hypoglycemic you are, how much and how long you deviate from the diet and how conspicuous your symptoms are.

Q. How soon after starting the Krimmel Program can I expect to begin enjoying some benefits?

A. Often within 3–10 days you will see the lessening of the severity of some symptoms if not the total disappearance of some. In 30 days you will definitely see a change and for a full clear picture give yourself 90 days.

Q. What is the basis of the Krimmel Program?

A. 1. A diet without refined carbohydrates and no foods which contain a high amount of natural sugar such as dried fruits and some fruit juices (grape, apple, prune). Also no caffeine containing products (colas, coffee, tea, etc.) and tobacco.
2. Exercise.
3. Proper rest.
4. Fun and laughter.

Q. What is a diet analysis?

A. It is a review of what you eat in relation to refined carbohydrates, complex carbohydrates, proteins and fats.

Q. Isn't it more expensive to buy all unrefined food products than refined foods such as macaroni, spaghetti and white flour etc.?

A. No. Usually the more unrefined a food is, the longer it takes to be metabolized and therefore it stays with you longer and you do not become hungry as soon as you do after eating refined foods which are metabolized much more quickly. A smaller amount of unrefined foods will satisfy you more than a larger amount of refined foods. Compare eating a piece of fresh fruit to the same amount of canned fruit. In the end, in my opinion, you will be buying less food but of a higher quality and spending no more money. Also the higher quality foods you eat the less chance you have of tooth problems and other degenerative diseases which lead to medical expenses.

Q. Why is exercise so very important?

A. In many ways exercise is more important than the proper food. Food you can live without for many days but you can only live a few minutes without oxygen. But, you say, as long as I am breathing I am getting oxygen. True, but the higher the level of oxygen your body receives the better you feel and function. When you exercise, brisk walking for example, you breathe deeper and take in more oxygen, your heart beats faster and pumps the oxygen carrying blood through your body to all your cells so then things can function at their optimum level. Exercise tones up muscles, improves digestion and improves your circulation. Have you ever said after a day of physical activity, "Boy, am I tired, but it is a *good* tired feeling." The reason it is a good tired feeling rather than the tired feeling you get from sedentary work is that the physical work increased your blood circulation and carried more oxygen to your cells so they can function at their highest level.

Q. Why does LBS cause such things as visual problems and aching muscles which would seem so unrelated to each other?

A. Since your body's cells need blood sugar for energy, they aren't able to function to their best ability when there is not enough available to them. The retina of the eye can use *only* glucose for energy so when there isn't enough glucose available you have visual disturbances. When the muscles don't have enough glucose to do the work you want them to do, they hurt.

Q. Are there any quick and easy solutions to any of the low blood sugar symptoms?

A. Yes, headaches can usually be relieved by eating 4 to 6 ounces of plain yogurt plus lying down for a short time. Also sleeping difficulties can usually be helped by eating plain yogurt immediately before retiring and again if you awaken during the night. (see chapter 6, Vital Snacks section)

Q. Is it valuable for low blood sufferers to learn about food composition, and if so where can this information be found?

A. You may order this information from us, see back of book.

RECIPES

If interested in additional recipes, order our Low Blood Sugar Cookbook. See order form in back of book.

Following are a few recipes we have found enjoyable.

"OK" Oatmeal (2 servings)

1½ Cups boiling water
¼ teaspoon salt
⅔ Cup rolled oats

½ Cup unpeeled tart apple, chopped
1 teaspoon cinnamon

Stir oats into boiling salted water, add apples and cinnamon.

Cook 5 minutes or longer, stirring occasionally.

Cover, remove from heat and let stand a few minutes.

Serve with cream or milk and a pat of butter.

Healthy Hot Cakes (3–4 servings)

3 eggs
3 Tablespoons vegetable oil or melted butter
1 Cup milk

1 Cup oat flour
¼ Cup soy flour
¼ teaspoon salt
3 teaspoons baking powder

In a bowl combine eggs, oil, and milk. In a small bowl mix dry ingredients together and add to liquids. Mix thoroughly.

Spoon small amount on to hot griddle, bake until bubbly on top and underside nicely browned. Turn and bake till other side browned.

Serve with unsweetened applesauce and cinnamon or pureed peaches.

Pat's 3 Grain Bread (makes 2 loaves)

Have all ingredients at room temperature or slightly warmer.

Stir together in large mixing bowl:
  3 Cups whole wheat flour
  2 pkgs. yeast
  ⅔ Cup powdered milk
  2 tsp. salt

Add:
  ⅓ Cup oil or softened butter
  2 eggs
  2 Cups very warm water (120°)

Beat 5–10 minutes at medium speed of electric mixer.

Mix together and stir in by hand:
  6 Tbs. soy flour
  1 Cup rye flour
  1 ¼ Cups oat flour

Stir in:
  1 Cup oat flour
  1 Cup whole wheat flour

Sprinkle 1 Cup whole wheat flour on kneading surface and turn out dough onto it.

Oil your hands and begin kneading with fingertips until dough stiffens up.

Knead 5–10 minutes or until dough is smooth and elastic, add additional whole wheat flour as necessary.

Cover with plastic wrap and folded tea towel.

Let rest 20 minutes.

Punch down by kneading a few times.

Divide into 2 equal parts, and roll out each into about a 9″ × 12″ shape.

Roll up toward you, sealing edges well.

Place seam down in 9¾″ × 5¾″ × 2¾″ bread pans, well greased.

Cover with plastic wrap and refrigerate from 2–24 hours.

Bake at will.

Remove from refrigerator about 10 minutes before baking.

Uncover and puncture any air bubbles.

Bake at 350° 35–45 minutes.

Remove from pans and allow to cool on rack—and enjoy!

Lunchy Munchy Pizza

Sliced whole wheat or rye bread   Jarlsberg cheese
Spaghetti sauce   Parmesan cheese
Cheddar cheese

Toast bread, spread sauce on toast, place one layer of cheddar and one layer of Jarlsberg cheese, cover with spaghetti sauce, sprinkle on Parmesan cheese, place under broiler until cheese melts and is bubbly. May add slices of green pepper and/or mushroom slices.

Super Eggplant Parmesan (6 servings)

1 eggplant—1½ lbs.
2 eggs, beaten
1¼ Cups wheat germ
¾ tsp. salt
½ tsp. pepper

15 ounce can tomato sauce
1 tsp. basil
½ tsp. oregano
1 lb. mozzarella cheese, sliced
½ Cup Parmesan cheese, grated

Wash eggplant and cut crosswise into ½ inch slices.

Dip slices of eggplant into eggs.

Coat slices with mixture of wheat germ, salt and pepper.

Place slices on plate and refrigerate ½ hour.

Broil eggplant until brown on both sides.

Heat tomato sauce, basil and oregano.

Spread small amount of sauce in greased 12 × 8 × 2 inch baking dish.

Place ½ eggplant in bottom of dish.

Place ½ mozzarella cheese next.

Cover with ½ remaining sauce.

Sprinkle ½ parmesan cheese over sauce.

Repeat layers.

Bake at 350° for about 30 mintues or until bubbly.

Neat Sweet and Sour Tofu and Vegetables (serves 4)

Combine the following six items
and set aside.
1 Tbs. cider vinegar
6 Tbs. water
¼ Cup pineapple juice
2 Tbs. soy sauce
¼–½ tsp. ginger
dash pepper

2 Tbs. oil
1 medium onion, chopped
2 carrots, sliced thinly, diagonally
¾ lb. tofu, cut into chunks
1 green pepper, chopped
¼ tsp. salt
⅔ Cup pineapple chunks (in own
juice) with juice

Heat oil in a wok or large skillet over high heat.

Add onion and stir until strong odor begins to leave, add carrots and stir.

Add tofu and stir until lightly browned, add peppers and salt.

Stir about 1 minute, then cover, reduce heat to medium and cook until carrots are partly cooked.

Add pineapple and liquid mixture, cook covered for about 10 minutes.

Serve with brown rice if desired.

No-Dough Zucchini Lasagna (10–12 servings)

2 ½–3 lbs. large zucchini, washed
    and scrubbed
1 quart spaghetti sauce (without
    any type of sugar added)
1 Cup wheat germ
2 lbs. ricotta cheese
4 eggs, beaten

2 Tbs. chopped parsley
½ tsp. oregano
½ tsp. basil
Salt and pepper as desired
1 Cup grated Parmesan cheese
1 lb. mozzarella cheese, grated

Trim ends of zucchini and slice (unpeeled) into long thin slices.

Combine ricotta cheese, eggs, parsley, seasonings and ½ Cup Parmesan cheese and 6 Tbs. wheat germ.

1) Spoon into a 9″ × 14″ × 2″ pan a thin layer of spaghetti sauce.
2) Sprinkle ¼ Cup wheat germ over sauce.
3) Place layer of zucchini, with slices side by side over wheat germ.
4) Spread ½ ricotta cheese mixture over zucchini.
5) Spread ½ lb. grated mozzarella cheese next.
6) Spread layer tomato sauce.
7) Layer zucchini (keep few slices for top).
8) Spread rest of ricotta mixture.
9) Spread layer of tomato sauce (keep small amount for top).
10) Place few slices of zucchini down center of dish.
11) Sprinkle rest of mozzarella cheese and spaghetti sauce on top.
12) combine remaining wheat germ and Parmesan cheese and
       sprinkle over top.

Bake at 350° for about 1 hour or until top browned.

Let stand for 20 minutes before serving.

Ideal for cooking a day ahead of when needed.

Simple Applesauce

May use any type of apple but tart ones are preferable.

Wash apples and remove stems. Do not peel or remove seeds.

Cut into ¼s and put in a pan with enough water to cover bottom to prevent sticking or burning.

Bring to a boil and cook until apples are soft.

Put apples through a food mill, do not add sugar of any kind.

May add cinnamon if desired.

Keeps in refrigerator for about one week or freeze for longer storage.

Dessert Fruit Gelatin

Sprinkle 1 envelope of Knox unflavored gelatin on ¼ Cup of cold water in a saucepan.

Heat over low heat and stir constantly for about 1–3 minutes until gelatin dissolves.

Pour into 1 ½ Cup any permitted juice and stir.

Place in refrigerator to set.

If desired, may add some sliced peaches, bananas, oranges, pineapple or berries when gelatin is partially set.

Puffy Clouds Peach Pie

Sprinkle 2 envelopes of unflavored Knox gelatin on ½ Cup of cold water in saucepan.

Heat over low heat for 1–3 minutes stirring constantly until gelatin is dissolved.

Pour into 3 Cups fresh squeezed orange juice and stir.

Refrigerate until partially set.

Whip ½ Cup of heavy whipping cream until stiff, add 1 tsp. vanilla and 1 Tbs. thawed pineapple juice and whip till forms peaks.

Fold whipped cream into partially set gelatin.

Have bottom of 9″ glass pie plate covered with sliced peaches and pour gelatin mixture over them.

Refrigerate until completely set.

Better if made a day ahead.

Kiddie Pops—Summer Treat

Use any type of pure unsweetened fruit juice, add a small amount of water so it freezes harder.

Pour into popsicle molds or 3 oz. paper cups, when partially frozen put in stick or plastic spoon.

To serve peel away paper cup when completely frozen.

Great Strawberry Shake

2 Cups milk
2 Cups fresh or frozen strawberries (not in syrup)
1 tsp. vanilla
½ Cups non-instant dry milk

Blend all together in blender, add 3–4 ice cubes and blend until very cold. Serving = ¾–1 cup

BIBLIOGRAPHY

Abrahamson, E.M. and Pezet, A.W.: BODY, MIND, AND SUGAR. Pyramid Paperbacks, New York, 1971

Adams, Ruth and Murray, Frank: IS LOW BLOOD SUGAR MAKING YOU A NUTRITIONAL CRIPPLE? Larchmont Books, New York, 1975

Blevimand, Margo and Ginder, Geri: THE LOW BLOOD SUGAR COOKBOOK. Doubleday and Co., Inc., Garden City, N.Y., 1973

Brennan, R.O. with Mulligan, William C.: NUTRIGENTICS. Signet, New York, 1975

Cheraskin, E. M.D., et al.: PSYCHODIETETICS. Bantam Books, New York, 1974

Duffy, William: SUGAR BLUES. Warner Books, Inc., New York, 1975

Goldbeck, David and Nikki: THE SUPERMARKET HANDBOOK. Plume Books, New York, 1973

Gray, Henry: GRAY'S ANATOMY. Lea and Febiger, Philadelphia, Pennsylvania, 1974

Guyton, Arthur C.: TEXTBOOK OF MEDICAL PHYSIOLOGY. W.B. Saunders Company, Philadelphia, Pennsylvania, 1981

Martin, Clement G.: LOW BLOOD SUGAR, THE HIDDEN MENACE OF HYPOGLYCEMIA. Arco Publishing Co., Inc., New York, 1976

Nutrition Search Inc.: NUTRITIONAL ALMANAC. McGraw-Hill, New York, 1975

Ross, Harvey: FIGHTING DEPRESSION. Larchmont Books, New York, 1975

Saunders, Jeraldine and Ross, Harvey: HYPOGLYCEMIA: THE DISEASE YOUR DOCTOR WON'T TREAT. Pinnacle Books, Inc., New York, 1980

Schauss, Alexander: DIET, CRIME AND DELINQUENCY. Parker House, 2340 Parker Street, Berkeley, California, 1980

Smith, Lendon: IMPROVING YOUR CHILD'S CHEMISTRY. Pocket Books, New York, 1977

Steincrohn, Peter: LOW BLOOD SUGAR. Henry Regnery Co., Chicago, 1972

Taber, Clarence Wilbur: TABER'S CYCLOPEDIC MEDICAL DICTIONARY. F.A. Davis Company, Philadelphia, Pennsylvania, 1981

Trotter, Robert J.: AGGRESSION: A WAY OF LIFE FOR THE QOLLA. Science News, February 3, 1973, p. 76

Weller, Charles and Boylan, Brian Richard: HOW TO LIVE WITH HYPOGLYCEMIA. Award Books, New York, 1975

Yudkin, John M.D.: SWEET AND DANGEROUS. Bantam Books, New York, 1972

GLOSSARY

ABSORPTION. The process by which nutrients are taken up by the intestines and passed into the blood stream.

ADRENAL GLAND. One located on top of each kidney, produces hormones essential to life, one being adrenalin.

ADRENALIN. Hormone produced by adrenal gland to prepare body for physical action, by increasing heart rate, diverting blood to the muscles, and stimulates liver to convert glycogen stored in the liver to glucose to be used for energy.

ALLERGY. Hypersensitivity by body tissues to a specific substance which is usually harmless such as dust, pollen, foods and animal fur. May cause inflammation of skin, nose and eyes, intestinal upset, wheezy breathing and headaches etc.

AMINO ACIDS. Organic compounds which are the building blocks of proteins. There are about 22 amino acids of which 9 are essential because they cannot be manufactured by the body so must be supplied adequately from the foods you eat.

ANXIETY. A feeling of apprehension from either a real or imagined threatening situation.

ARTERIES. The tubes which carry the blood away from the heart to all parts of the body.

ASSIMILATE. To absorb digested food into the system.

BLOOD. The fluid that circulates through the heart, arteries, veins and capillaries carrying nourishment and oxygen to the tissues and taking away waste and carbon dioxide.

BLOOD SUGAR. Sugar in the blood. Normal is 80–120 mg of glucose per 100 cc of blood.

BRAIN. Main organ of the nervous system, protected by the skull. Regulates all the body's responses, from basic movements to emotions and intelligence.

CAFFEINE. A stimulant and diuretic found in coffee, tea, colas, cocoa and chocolate.

CALORIES. Amount of chemical energy that is released as heat when food is metabolized.

CARBOHYDRATES. One of the three basic food materials containing only carbon, hydrogen and oxygen. The smallest carbohydrates are simple sugars which may join together to form larger molecules found in starches.

CELL. The basic and smallest functional and structural unit of all living forms.

CENTRAL NERVOUS SYSTEM (CNS). Brain, spinal cord and their nerves.

CHYME. The partially digested, semi-liquid mass into which food is converted by the gastric juices before it leaves the stomach.

CIRCULATORY SYSTEM. Transportation of blood by the arteries to all parts of the body and returned to the heart by the veins.

COLON. Part of the large intestine between the cecum and rectum, divided into the ascending, the transverse and the descending colon.

DIABETES. Condition resulting from the body's faulty utilization of glucose. The blood glucose rises above the normal level.

DIGESTION. The breakdown of food by mechanical and chemical processes brought about by enzymes secreted in the stomach and intestine. The large molecules are reduced to small molecules which are absorbed through the intestinal wall and carried in the blood to the liver and other parts of the body to be utilized.

DUODENUM. The first part of the small intestine, lies between the stomach and jejunum. The digestive juices from the pancreas and bile from the liver enter the duodenum.

ENDOCRINE GLANDS. Glands which secrete their product into the blood stream. They secrete hormones which affect body functions.

ENDOCRINOLOGIST. One who treats conditions related to the endocrine system.

ENZYME. A protein substance which brings about chemical changes.

ESOPHAGUS. Tube which carries food from the back of the throat to the stomach. Muscular contractions of the esophagus wall push food and drink down the esophagus.

ESSENTIAL AMINO ACIDS. The nine amino acids that cannot be made by the body. They are Listidine, Isoleucine, Leucine, Lysine, Total S-containing amino acids (includes methionine), Total aromatic amino acids (includes Phenylalanine), Threonine, Tryptophan, Valine.

FAST ACTING CARBOHYDRATE. Carbohydrates which are broken down very rapidly into glucose. These are usually refined carbohydrates which include white flour and all types of sugars.

FAT. One of the main types of food we eat, provides richer source of energy than carbohydrates. Fat is stored in the adipose tissue of the body.

FAT SOLUBLE VITAMIN. Vitamin which is able to dissolve in fats or oils.

FRUCTOSE. One of the sugars in fruits.

GLUCAGON. A hormone secreted by the pancreas that increases the level of glucose in the blood.

GLUCOSE. A simple sugar and the simplest form in which a carbohydrate is assimilated in the body; blood sugar. A major source of energy for all human cells.

GLYCOGEN. The form in which glucose is stored in the body.

GOITER. An enlargement of the thyroid gland.

HEMOGLOBIN. The part of the red blood cell which contains iron and protein.

HEREDITY. The passing of characteristics (color of hair and eyes, tendency for certain diseases or conditions) from parent to child through the genes.

HORMONE. A chemical substance secreted into the blood stream by an endocrine gland. It acts on an organ in another part of the body.

HYPERINSULINISM. Too much insulin in blood stream. A term sometimes used interchangeably with hypoglycemia.

HYPOGLYCEMIA. Too little glucose in the blood stream for the body's cells to function properly.

INORGANIC. Substance occurring independently of living things.

INSULIN. A hormone secreted by the pancreas which regulates the metabolism of sugar.

INTESTINE. Digestive tract from stomach to anus.

IODINE. Necessary for the development and functioning of the thyroid gland and to prevent goiter.

ISLETS OF LANGERHANS. Collection of cells in the pancreas which secrete insulin and glucagon.

LACTASE. An enzyme secreted in the small intestine which breaks down lactose (milk sugar).

LACTOSE. A carbohydrate; milk sugar, composed of glucose and galactose, two simple sugars.

LARGE INTESTINE. The part of the digestive tract between the small intestine and the anus, approximately 5 feet long and 2½ inches in diameter. It is divided into 3 parts—the colon, the cecum and the rectum. Materials from small intestine go into the large intestine where much of the material's water is absorbed and then the semisolid waste is stored until passed from the body as feces.

LEGUMES. Plants with seed-containing pods that are used as food.

LIVER. The largest organ in the body, some of its functions are: bile production, synthesis of proteins and carbohydrates, storage of glucose, minerals and vitamins and breaking down of poisons, one being alcohol.

METABOLISM. The chemical process by which food is changed into energy, and new material is assimilated for the repair and replacement of tissues.

MINERAL. Nutrients in the body and food of inorganic substances such as calcium, phosphorus, potassium etc.

MOLECULE. The smallest unit into which a substance can be divided and retain its chemical identity.

NERVES. Bands of nerve tissue that conduct information to or from the brain and any part of the body.

NERVOUS SYSTEM. System of nerve cells consisting of the brain, cranial nerves, spinal cord, spinal nerves, autonomic ganglia, ganglionated trunks and nerves, maintaining the vital function of reception and response to stimuli.

NUTRIENT. A basic substance required by a living thing to maintain life, health and reproduction.

ORGAN. A structure of the body that has some special purpose such as the liver, heart, brain and lungs.

OXIDATION. A change occurring because of oxygen chemically combining with another substance.

OXYGEN. A tasteless, colorless, odorless gas essential to the energy producing processes of all living things by which food materials are burned up by oxidation.

PANCREAS. A large gland just below the stomach which pours digestive juices into the small intestine. Also secretes insulin and glucagon into the blood stream to regulate glucose metabolism.

PITUITARY GLAND. A small gland in the brain which secretes substances necessary for basic life processes.

PORTAL VEIN. The large blood vessel which transports nutrients, that have come from the veins of the stomach and intestine, to the liver.

PROTEIN. One of the three basic food materials which is essential for the building and repair of body tissue. It is made up of long chains of 22 amino acids, of which 9 are essential because they cannot be manufactured by the body so they must be obtained from the foods you eat. In order for the body to utilize protein it must be a "complete protein" which means all nine essential amino acids must be present in your meal. They can come from combining foods to make up the 9 essential amino acids.

PTYALIN. Enzyme, found in saliva, necessary for carbohydrate breakdown.

PULSE. The periodic expansion of the arteries caused by the heart pushing (pumping) additional blood into the arteries.

RECOMMENDED DAILY ALLOWANCE (RDA). The amount of nutrients suggested by the National Research Council as being necessary to maintain life processes in most healthy persons.

RESPIRATION. The act of breathing. Process by which oxygen enters the lungs and the waste products of water and carbon dioxide leave the lungs.

RESPIRATORY SYSTEM. The system of the body related to breathing, including the mouth, nasal passages, trachea (windpipe) which divides into 2 bronchi (tubes) leading to the lungs.

RETINA. Lining at the back of the eye, the perceptive structure on which light rays focus and form an image.

RHEUMATIC FEVER. Disease in which there is fever, swollen and aching joints and the heart valves frequently become inflamed.

RICKETS. Disease in children in which the bones become soft and often bend. Caused by lack of vitamin D.

SALIVARY GLANDS. Six glands in the mouth that secrete saliva, watery fluid containing digestive enzymes.

SCURVY. Condition caused by vitamin C deficiency, gums swell and bleed.

SLOW ACTING CARBOHYDRATE. Natural, unrefined carbohydrates; all fresh fruits, vegetables and grains.

SPINAL CORD. An extension of the brain filling ⅔ of the canal running through the spine. It is a column of nervous tissue capable of initiating reflex responses and contains nerve tracts carrying impulses to and from the brain. There are 31 pairs of nerves going out from the spinal cord to all areas of the body.

STARCH. Complex carbohydrate which is broken down into glucose during digestion. Contained in such foods as potatoes, corn and whole grain cereals.

STIMULANT. Any agent that temporarily increases functional activity. Examples are caffeine and nicotine.

STOMACH. A large muscular bag below the diaphragm which receives the food from the esophagus. It mixes the food with digestive enzymes and acids secreted from its walls. It churns and softens the food particles and passes them into the small intestine.

STRESS. Anything (physical or mental) that places unnecessary strain on the glandular or nervous system of the body.

SUGARS. Simple carbohydrates such as glucose, lactose, maltose and sucrose.

SUPPLEMENT. Nutrients taken in addition to regular diet.

SYMPTOM. Anything that indicates a body disorder.

TASTE BUDS. Clusters of nerve cell receptors on the tongue that respond to sweetness, sourness, bitterness and saltiness.

THYROID GLAND. Two lobes lying on either side of the trachea (windpipe) which are stimulated by a pituitary hormone to produce thyroxin which increases the rate of the body's cells activity.

TRACE MINERALS. Elements present in minute quantities which are essential to the life of an organism.

VEINS. Blood vessels which carry blood from the body's tissues to the heart. Valves are in the veins which prevent the back flow of blood and aid the muscular activity of the body to push the blood toward the heart.

VERTIGO. Dizzy feeling; feeling that everything around one is whirling about.

VITAMINS. Nutrients found in foods which perform specific and necessary functions in the body.

WATER SOLUBLE VITAMIN. Vitamin able to be dissolved in water.

INDEX

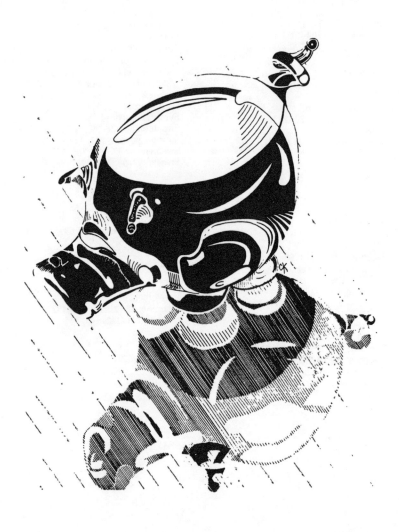

Reflections of a pig

Charles A. Krimmel

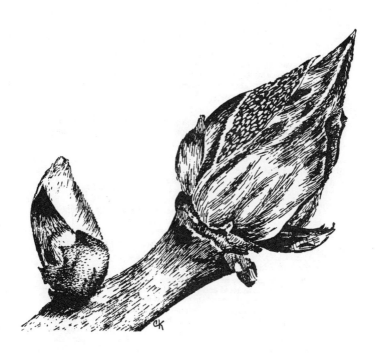

New Life

Charles A. Krimmel

To order, send note or copy of order form with payment

ORDER YOUR COPY(S) TODAY!

Please send:

_____ **THE LOW BLOOD SUGAR HANDBOOK (Revised Edition)**
copy(s) *By Edward & Patricia Krimmel* $12.95
Highly praised by Harvey Ross, M.D., this is a new upscaled approach
to the diagnosis and treatment of hypoglycemia (low blood sugar), written with the insight and practicality that only a sufferer could have, but
backed up by meticulous research and medical accuracy. The book of
solutions! 192 pages

_____ **THE LOW BLOOD SUGAR COOKBOOK**
copy(s) *By Patricia & Edward Krimmel* $12.95
A very special collection of over 200 sugarless natural food recipes. Snacks
to gourmet dishes designed specifically for the hypoglycemic, but which
everyone can enjoy and are also valuable to diabetics and weight watch-
ers. No artificial sweeteners or white flour are used in the recipes. Only
fruit and fruit juices are used as sweeteners. 192 pages

_____ **THE LOW BLOOD SUGAR CASSETTE**
copy(s) *By Edward & Patricia Krimmel* $9.95
A one (1) hour interview conceptualizing many of the most important
questions and answers pertaining to low blood sugar. Receive the feeling
of personal contact with the authors.

_____ **COMPOSITION OF FOODS BOOKLET** $4.50
copy(s) Allows you to determine:
• which foods are most beneficial for you
• which foods are low in fat for losing weight and reducing your cholesterol count
• the amount of calories you are eating. Booklet lists the amount of
  calories, carbohydrate, protein, fat, (total, saturated, mono-
  unsaturated, polyunsaturated) and cholesterol in the majority of foods.

_____ **CHOLESTEROL LOWERING AND CONTROLLING 3 WEEK**
copy(s) **PLAN: HANDBOOK & COOKBOOK**
By Patricia & Edward Krimmel $12.95
Tells how to be properly tested, finger stick is not test of choice. Do you
know which foods to avoid and why, and which foods to eat and why?
What about weight reduction? Do you want to understand how to lose
weight correctly and easily for a lifetime? Do you know which oils should
be used and which ones to avoid and how to decrease the amount of
saturated fat you eat? All these issues and many, many more are covered
in clear, easy to understand language for a lifetime of benefit. A physician
recommended book of vital information and tasty recipes.

Send check or money order to **Franklin Publishers, Box 1338, Bryn Mawr, PA 19010.** For
total order, include $2.00 for postage and handling or $3.00 for 1st class postage and
handling. PA residents, include state sales tax.

Orders outside of U.S. must be paid in U.S. dollars with a Postal Money Order.

Send to:

Mr./Ms. _____
(Print or type)

Address_____

City_____ State_____ Zip_____

Phone number _____
Price subject to change without notice.

ORDER YOUR COPY(S) TODAY!

__copy(s)__ THE LOW BLOOD SUGAR HANDBOOK (Revised edition) $12.95

__copy(s)__ THE LOW BLOOD SUGAR COOKBOOK $12.95

__copy(s)__ THE LOW BLOOD SUGAR CASSETTE (1 hour) . . . . $ 9.95

__copy(s)__ COMPOSITION OF FOODS BOOKLET . . . . $ 4.50

__copy(s)__ CHOLESTEROL LOWERING AND CONTROLLING
3 WEEK PLAN: HANDBOOK & COOKBOOK $12.95

Send check or money order to: Franklin Publishers, Box 1338, Bryn Mawr, PA 19010.
For total order, include $2.00 for postage and handling or $3.00 for 1st class postage
and handling.   PA residents, include state sales tax.

Orders outside of U.S. must be paid in U.S. dollars with a Postal Money Order.

Send to:

Mr./Ms. _____
(Print or type)

Address_____

City_____ State_____ Zip_____

Phone number _____

Price subject to change without notice.

ORDER YOUR COPY(S) TODAY!

__copy(s)__ THE LOW BLOOD SUGAR HANDBOOK (Revised edition) $12.95

__copy(s)__ THE LOW BLOOD SUGAR COOKBOOK $12.95

__copy(s)__ THE LOW BLOOD SUGAR CASSETTE (1 hour) . . . . $ 9.95

__copy(s)__ COMPOSITION OF FOODS BOOKLET . . . . $ 4.50

__copy(s)__ CHOLESTEROL LOWERING AND CONTROLLING
3 WEEK PLAN: HANDBOOK & COOKBOOK $12.95

Send check or money order to: Franklin Publishers, Box 1338, Bryn Mawr, PA 19010.
For total order, include $2.00 for postage and handling or $3.00 for 1st class postage
and handling.   PA residents, include state sales tax.

Orders outside of U.S. must be paid in U.S. dollars with a Postal Money Order.

Send to:

Mr./Ms. _____
(Print or type)

Address_____

City_____ State_____ Zip_____

Phone number _____

Price subject to change without notice.

ORDER YOUR COPY(S) TODAY!

_____ THE LOW BLOOD SUGAR HANDBOOK (Revised edition) $12.95
copy(s)

_____ THE LOW BLOOD SUGAR COOKBOOK $12.95
copy(s)

_____ THE LOW BLOOD SUGAR CASSETTE (1 hour) ....$ 9.95
copy(s)

_____ COMPOSITION OF FOODS BOOKLET ....$ 4.50
copy(s)

_____ CHOLESTEROL LOWERING AND CONTROLLING
copy(s) 3 WEEK PLAN: HANDBOOK & COOKBOOK $12.95

Send check or money order to: **Franklin Publishers, Box 1338, Bryn Mawr, PA 19010.**
For total order, include $2.00 for postage and handling or $3.00 for 1st class postage
and handling.   PA residents, include state sales tax.

Orders outside of U.S. must be paid in U.S. dollars with a Postal Money Order.

Send to:

Mr./Ms. _____
          (Print or type)

Address_____

City_____ State_____ Zip_____

Phone number _____
                        Price subject to change without notice.

ORDER YOUR COPY(S) TODAY!

_____ THE LOW BLOOD SUGAR HANDBOOK (Revised edition) $12.95
copy(s)

_____ THE LOW BLOOD SUGAR COOKBOOK $12.95
copy(s)

_____ THE LOW BLOOD SUGAR CASSETTE (1 hour) ....$ 9.95
copy(s)

_____ COMPOSITION OF FOODS BOOKLET ....$ 4.50
copy(s)

_____ CHOLESTEROL LOWERING AND CONTROLLING
copy(s) 3 WEEK PLAN: HANDBOOK & COOKBOOK $12.95

Send check or money order to: **Franklin Publishers, Box 1338, Bryn Mawr, PA 19010.**
For total order, include $2.00 for postage and handling or $3.00 for 1st class postage
and handling.   PA residents, include state sales tax.

Orders outside of U.S. must be paid in U.S. dollars with a Postal Money Order.

Send to:

Mr./Ms. _____
          (Print or type)

Address_____

City_____ State_____ Zip_____

Phone number _____
                        Price subject to change without notice.

The authors encourage you to share with them any questions or insights you may have. A great amount of work still needs to be done in the study of low blood sugar and its effects. If an answer is desired, include a stamped, self addressed envelope. Please write to us c/o:

Franklin Publishers
P.O. Box 1338
Bryn Mawr, Pa. 19010

ABOUT THE AUTHORS

Edward and Patricia Krimmel and their son, Charles, live in the suburbs of Philadelphia, Pa.

Patricia and Edward Krimmel are medical researchers and writers who have a special aptitude and spirit for relating very well to those trying to solve health problems. Because of their backgrounds, they are especially well equipped to write and design books dealing with solutions rather than simply talking about the problem. They are the authors of two other books; *The Low Blood Sugar Cookbook* and *The Cholesterol Lowering and Controlling Handbook and Cookbook*.

Pat has her BSN from the University of Pennsylvania, has worked in childbirth education, public health and has been Maternal and Infant Care Coordinator at the Medical College of Pennsylvania.

Ed has his degree in Social Science from Saint Joseph's University, is Director of Help, The Institute For Body Chemistry, and does nutritional counseling.

The knowledge for this book is a direct result of the victimizing and suffering Ed and Pat experienced due to Ed's having low blood sugar, in addition to the reading, studying and research required.

The inspiration for the book came from having worked with low blood sugar victims in helping them understand and regulate their blood sugar.

COMMUNITY SUPPORT GROUP

If interested in having a self help support group started in your community or locating one already established, mail your name, address and phone number to: Franklin Publishers, Box 1338, Bryn Mawr, PA 19010. Include a self addressed, stamped envelope.

NEWSLETTER! NEWSLETTER! NEWSLETTER!

How would you like to receive current information in the world of body chemistry, nutrition, biochemistry, LBS, PMS, well-being, and so on? Send a self addressed, stamped envelope to: Franklin Publishers, Box 1338, Bryn Mawr, PA 19010.